Vaccines:

Point by Point

The hidden information you need for making one of the most important decisions for your child (and you).

Dr. Michael Nichols

Printed in the United States of America
First Printing, 2026
ISBN 9798218877316

GTH Press
Cincinnati, Ohio
www.DoctorMichaelNichols.com

Table of Contents

Foreword

In an era where medical decisions are increasingly influenced by mandates, media narratives, and institutional pressures, this book stands as a vital call to reclaim one of our most fundamental human rights: the right to personal choice and bodily autonomy. As a scientist and a father, I want to encourage all individuals making vaccine choices to understand as completely as possible the risks versus benefits of vaccination. This collection of "Points"—from the history of vaccines to conflicts of interest, media bias, ingredient concerns, and specific case studies like chickenpox, autism links, and the SARS-CoV-2 response—offers a comprehensive, unflinching examination of a subject too often shrouded in dogma.

Dr. Nichol's journey, beginning as a chiropractic student in the late 1990s and evolving through decades of research and clinical experience, mirrors the path many parents and individuals take when they first encounter doubts about the vaccine paradigm. What starts as a quest for balanced information reveals layers of complexity: the exponential growth in vaccine schedules since the 1980s, the removal of manufacturer liability in 1986, and the capture of regulatory bodies by industry interests. These are not mere conspiracy theories but documented realities, drawn from historical records, scientific studies, and public data. The book doesn't demand you reject vaccines outright; instead, it insists you understand them fully—their origins in a time of poor sanitation and woefully incomplete medical knowledge, their evolution into a liability-free enterprise, and their real-world implications for health.

At the heart of this work is the principle of bodily autonomy. No one—not governments, corporations, or even well-meaning experts—should have the authority to compel medical interventions. Dr. Nichols eloquently argues that personal and medical freedom are cornerstones of a just society, echoing thinkers like Hiroko Mori who remind us that the right to say "no" is a human right. This isn't about selfishness; it's about sovereignty over one's own body and those of our children. In a world where outbreaks are often blamed on the unvaccinated (despite evidence showing vaccinated individuals can also spread disease), and where herd immunity is wielded as a moral cudgel (dissected in the book as a concept often misunderstood and misapplied), the book challenges us to prioritize individual rights over collective assumptions.

Equally crucial is the emphasis on understanding risks. Vaccines are not "perfectly safe," as Dr. Nichols meticulously details by presenting many peer-reviewed studies and real-world examples of adverse events. From the adjuvants and by-products in ingredients to the unstudied synergies in modern schedules, the author presents evidence that demands scrutiny. Comparative studies of vaccinated versus unvaccinated populations highlighted in the book reveal gaps in research that should alarm anyone committed to evidence-based medicine. Even controversial figures like Dr. Andrew Wakefield are appropriately reframed not as villains, but as symbols of how dissent is silenced through character assassination and censorship. And in the wake of the COVID-19 era, the book exposes how fear and false evidence can erode freedoms, urging us to learn from this "culmination of decades" of agenda-driven policies.

This isn't a polemic against science; it's a defense of it. True science thrives on questioning, not unquestioned authority. Dr. Nichols, often dismissed as "not a real doctor", brings a perspective outside the pharmaceutical echo chamber, enriched by pediatric training and self-study. By weighing risks versus benefits, the book uniquely equips readers to make decisions that align with their values and circumstances—whether for mild diseases like chickenpox or broader programs.

As you delve into these pages, remember: knowledge is the antidote to coercion. In a landscape where conflicts of interest abound and history is often rewritten by victors, this book empowers you to think critically, protect your autonomy, and advocate for transparency. Personal choice isn't a luxury; it's essential to human dignity. As the father of a vaccine-injured, adult son, I implore you to read with an open mind, question boldly, and choose wisely—for yourself, your family, and the future of informed health.

~Brain Hooker, PhD., Chief Scientific
Officer Children's Health Defense

Acknowledgements

Books are not made alone. Even if you do all of the research and all of the writing, it is difficult to complete without support and understanding from others. This is especially true of family. The ones you are with the most who not only see your hard work and give you encouragement, but also give tolerance to having to hear your constant thoughts, ideas, concerns, complaints, hopes, dreams and fears regarding the same subject over and over.

For this and many more reasons, I thank my wife for her support and encouragement through this process. Also my children (young adults), who never (mostly) complained of hearing their dad speak incessantly about vaccines over the years.

Finally, a special thank you to all of the warrior moms (and dads) who have given so much to the Health Freedom Movement (now MAHA) over the decades. Your work and sacrifices do not go unnoticed.

Introduction

My journey with vaccines began back in 1998 while still in chiropractic college. Contrary to popular opinion, chiropractors are not taught to be anti-vaccine while in college. The information I received while in chiropractic college was fairly balanced if not slightly pro-vaccine. However, in 1998, while still attending chiropractic college, I began a Fellowship in Pediatrics through the International Chiropractic Pediatrics Association. The program focused on many things related to caring for a pediatric population and the topic of vaccines was only a week's worth of information. This was, however, the first time I received the depth of information regarding vaccines from the perspective of questioning the narrative. The instructor was not trying to tell us what to think but instead was giving us information and evidence that was intended to make us think about vaccines with a critical mind. The information went contrary to what little I had already known about vaccines and it intrigued me. This information created an awareness that there was more to the story and made me want to know more.

The first book about vaccines that I read was A Shot in the Dark by Harris L. Coulter and Barbara Loe Fisher. For many, this was the book that led them down the rabbit hole. For me it was just interesting information, that is until I got married and the idea of having kids became a reality. The next book I read was The Vaccine Guide by Randall Neustaedter, OMD. This was the book that opened up Pandora's box for me.

The book set out the information regarding the pros and cons about vaccinating in a clear, concise way and then offered the reader to make up their own mind. This connected with me and led to over twenty years of investigating the subject of vaccines. Since that first discussion about vaccines back in 1998, I have read dozens of books and hundreds of research articles, attended dozens of lectures, met hundreds of families of vaccine injured children and taken the deepest of deep dives through the internet looking for everything I can about this topic of vaccines.

This topic has proved to be quite the eye-opener for me. The information I have uncovered over the past two decades (plus) has shown me not only the highly questionable history of vaccines (Point 2) and the dangers inherent in getting vaccinated (Point 7), but it also revealed the lengths at which the vaccine apologists will go to keep this program from being questioned. The sheer quantity of blatant censorship towards anyone who questions the vaccine program and the often brutal attacks made against the personalities and careers of those that "question the science" reveals the lengths that the vaccine apologists will go to silence any opposition. There have been many scientists, medical doctors, academics and journalists who have been censored, lost jobs or been effectively blacklisted in their careers. I go over much more of this in Point 3. Those involved in the vaccine program are so deeply invested at this point that they surely feel there is no turning back and that they must keep pushing forward despite the mounting evidence that their program is flawed and creating a potentially devastating situation for future generations. It is obvious to me that those at the core of this program would rather go down in flames fighting than give even one inch to those that question the validity of the vaccine program. And make no mistake, the number of people who are questioning the validity is growing every year. Especially since the debacles during Covid (Point 16).

One of the biggest issues surrounding the topic of vaccines is the lack of availability of balanced information for people to consume. This is why it states "hidden information" on the cover of this book. Typically the only message the average person gets is that vaccines are amazing and that the people who question them are crazy and not to be trusted.

The mere idea of questioning the vaccine program has become anathema to many in society. This is due to the constant, pervasive brain-washing that we get regarding vaccines. This has become progressively worse since the early 2000's to now. It certainly feels as though our government agencies and the media have both been captured by the pharmaceutical companies and act in complete concert to ensure that no one can question the Holy Grail/Cash Cow that is the vaccine program.

This lack of balanced information became very evident anytime a conversation regarding vaccines would arise. Although I knew that the points I was bringing up in these conversations could be backed up with research or other documentation, many of those whom I had these discussions with had no knowledge of this information and would continue to put forth the talking points from the CDC, ignoring or denying any of the points that I would bring up. The topic of vaccines is not a simple conversation to have. There are so many points that need to be understood to get the full picture and each of these points need their own research to understand them. Many people will not be willing to go to the lengths necessary to understand these individual points. Also, if you do a basic search online for the information all you are getting is a cultivated list that reflects what the CDC and the pharmaceutical companies wish you to see. To get to the real story you must be willing to do the deep dive. It was with this understanding that I set out to write this book. I wanted to explore what I considered the main points regarding vaccines in a concise, easy to read way so that those who need to get the "big picture" could do so without having to do 20 years worth of investigation. Each Point in this book is jam packed with research. Everything I state in this book is backed up and cited so that you can be sure that this is not a matter of personal opinion but instead cited so that you can look up the research and information for yourself to see where the truth lies. As with any issue, the individual should be able to look at both sides and then make up their own mind as to the direction they will take. That is not an easy task with the topic of vaccines. My hope is that the information that is contained in this book will help others to see the other side of the vaccine story that so many do not want you to see. Only then can a true informed decision be made.

Point Number One: Personal Freedom/Medical Freedom

"There are so many people who have suffered side effects from vaccination. All we are asking is to establish the right to say 'no.' The right to choose should be recognized as a fundamental human right."
-Hiroko Mori, former head of the infectious disease section at the Japanese Institute of Public Health

Over the past two decades, I have given many seminars regarding vaccines and their inherent risks. My seminars have always been created to help inform the audience of the salient information on vaccines so that they could be better able to make a more informed choice. My point has never been to force my point of view or to tell someone that they should do exactly as I do. My understanding has always been that it is better to make informed decisions and to not follow advice blindly, especially with something as important as injecting chemical or pharmaceutical agents into your child's or your own body. I have always believed that this idea of being able to make these decisions without penalty or coercion would be perceived as common sense to every individual listening. However, to my surprise, there have been many who do not seem to think so.

In every vaccine seminar I have given, I have always covered a variety of points: history, ingredients, dangers, etc... most of which I will cover in this book as well. The one topic I never really spent much time on however was medical/bodily autonomy. I simply never thought of it as an issue to be discussed, because it seemed to me to be a given. Who would ever argue against a person's right to choose what is best for their own body? Over the past several years that is proving to be a very large and growing falsehood. This particular topic has now become, more and more, the center point of my discussions regarding vaccines. Regardless of the questionable ingredients found in vaccines, the dubious history and the motivations of the vaccine companies; the bottom line for all of us should be the simple fact that it is your body (or your child's body) and should therefore be your choice. No one should be able to force you or your children to partake in a medical procedure unless you agree to it. This may sound simplistic but that is because it is this simple and should be this simple.

In the field of medicine, there is ample evidence to be found to show that patient autonomy in making medical decisions is paramount to good medical practice. A research paper written in the journal Cardiology in the Young entitled, "Respect for Patient Autonomy as a Medical Virtue," stated, "Respect for patient autonomy is an important and indispensable principle in the ethical practice of clinical medicine. Legal tenets recognise the centrality of this principle and the inherent right of patients of sound mind - properly informed - to make their own personal medical decisions."(1) If you were to do a search for the "Four Pillars of Medical Ethics," you would find dozens of references to a set of principles that were created to help guide medical professionals to make the best decisions for their patients. "Four commonly accepted principles of health care ethics, excerpted from Beauchamp and Childress (2008), include the:"

1. Principle of respect for autonomy
2. Principle of nonmaleficence
3. Principle of beneficence
4. Principle of justice.

The first principle, the Respect for Autonomy, states: "Any notion of moral decision-making assumes that rational agents are involved in making informed and voluntary decisions. In health care decisions, our respect for the autonomy of the patient would, in common parlance, imply that the patient has the capacity to act intentionally, with understanding, and without controlling influences that would mitigate against a free and voluntary act."(2) Catch the usage of the words "informed and voluntary decisions." This first principle tells the medical practitioner that it is the patient's decision to agree or disagree with the doctor's medical advice or opinion. In fact this principle goes a step further and insists there should be no "controlling influences."

Another famous document that could be applied in these circumstances is the Nuremberg Code. The Nuremberg Code was created in 1947 in response to Nazi experimentations. The first of these codes states:

1. The voluntary consent of the human subject is absolutely essential.

This means that the "person involved should have legal capacity to give consent; should be so situated as to be able to exercise free power of choice, without the intervention of any element of force, fraud, deceit, duress, overreaching, or other ulterior form of constraint or coercion; and should have sufficient knowledge and comprehension of the elements of the subject matter involved as to enable him to make an understanding and enlightened decision."(3) It could be argued that the Nuremberg Codes were created to give ethical guidelines for medical experimentation and not for everyday medical decisions. However, I would in turn argue that the case could be made that the concept of vaccination is in itself a form of experimentation and therefore these codes could and would still apply. After you have read all of the Points in this book you can then ask yourself if you have ever had "sufficient knowledge and comprehension of the elements of the subject matter involved as to enable him (or her) to make an understanding and enlightened decision." I do not think that the average individual has been given proper information to be able to state this.

Well known legal expert (but in no way a vaccine expert) Alan Dershowitz says that when it comes to the topic of vaccines, we have no freedom of choice. When asked on a television program whether "the government has a right to endanger" people who may have an adverse reaction to a vaccine by forcing them to take it, Dershowitz responded by stating, "The Supreme Court has said yes, and if the case came to the Supreme Court today, they would say yes, it would either be 9-0 or 8-1," Dershowitz responded. "It is not a debatable issue constitutionally. Look, they have a right to draft you and put your life in danger to help the country. The police power of the state is very considerable." "Dershowitz added that he agrees with the "moral argument" that no one should be subject to a vaccine that has not been fully vetted on the chance it could help other people and noted that he wouldn't want people to submit to a vaccine unless it is proven safe."(4) There are several points worth looking at in Mr. Dershowitz response, are vaccines "fully vetted," "are they proven safe" and the idea of the country "having a right to draft you."

Let's look first at drafting individuals for war as an example of the government's ability to force you into doing something dangerous. According to the Selective Service System, "once a man gets a notice that he has been found qualified for military service, he has the opportunity to make a claim for classification as a conscientious objector (CO)." Who can apply to be a conscientious objector? Anyone who has, "Beliefs which qualify a registrant for CO status may be religious in nature, but don't have to be. Beliefs may be moral or ethical; however, a man's reasons for not wanting to participate in a war must not be based on politics, expediency, or self-interest." The person who then qualifies as a CO must then serve in some type of "alternative service." All of these alternative services are non-life threatening.(5) So the argument that Mr. Dershowitz makes implying that the government can put your life in danger is not quite true. Even in the process of drafting for a war, our government must allow individuals the opportunity to "opt out" of placing their lives in danger. As for his other two points (or more appropriately, assumptions) regarding vaccines being "fully vetted" and "proven safe" I will attempt to answer them in a different section of this book. Suffice it to say for now that the answer to both of these points is...not so much.

Most parents believe that in order for their children to attend public school they must be vaccinated. I have had conversations with literally hundreds of individuals who have never even heard that there are exemptions to get out of vaccinating their children if they wish to and still be able to enroll them into public school. Schools do not give out information about their state's exemptions when they send out notices of vaccines required. Currently in the United States we have three types of exemptions available that parents can choose from to not have their children vaccinated. These exemptions, depending on which state you live in, are either Philosophical (I don't want it), Religious (my religious beliefs says no) or Medical (I, or a sibling, have had a past reaction to a vaccine).(6) So, similar to drafting someone for war, the government has given its citizens the ability to "opt out" of placing their lives in danger through the injection of vaccines. Upon hearing this information you could make the argument that this entire discussion of medical freedom is a moot point. A person might say, We have exemptions so why are you getting yourself all worked up over nothing? That is a great question. To understand why medical freedom/bodily autonomy is so important you must understand the political environment we are currently living in and the changes that have been occurring around this topic.

Beginning around 2015, a very strong push to remove all exemptions for children began taking place. California was the epicenter of this movement and as a result, they took away both the philosophical and religious exemptions. New York followed soon after, removing both the philosophical and religious exemptions as well. Very quickly Maine, West Virginia and Mississippi also removed both of these exemptions. This will make five states that only allow medical exemption, at the time of this writing. Twenty-nine other states have never had the philosophical exemptions, which allow you to deny vaccines simply because it is your right to decide what goes into your body. (7) There are also multiple states currently with bills in their state legislature with the objective of removing both philosophical and religious exemptions. So at least they are giving you the ability to use a medical exemption, right? The thing that must be understood about the medical exemption is that to be eligible it must be proven that you or a very close relative has had a severe reaction caused by a particular vaccine. This is next to impossible to achieve as proving vaccine injury is incredibly difficult and finding a medical professional who is willing to sign off on this exemption is equally difficult. Finding a medical doctor who is open to the possibility that a vaccine may have caused your child's injury is like finding a medical doctor who is more likely to tell you to take supplements than to prescribe you drugs, possible but certainly not probable. Medical doctors as a whole are taught to believe that vaccines are not the cause of problems but are the cure to ills. They are led to believe that there is no evidence to show that they are anything but good. Unless you can find an MD who is willing to scour the literature to educate themselves, that viewpoint will not change.

And what if this is a child's first vaccine? The medical exemption essentially says you must get the vaccine and have a severe reaction first before you can begin requesting to not have future shots. This makes this exemption, for all intents and purposes, useless. Taking away the philosophical and religious exemptions and leaving parents with only the medical exemption is essentially the same as taking away all of our rights to bodily autonomy when it comes to vaccination. Add to this that the average individual is not even aware that any of these exemptions even exist. As I previously mentioned, most individuals I have spoken with are not aware that you can choose to not vaccinate. I have even spoken with medical doctors who did not seem to understand that exemptions existed. This speaks to the lack of information being given to the public in regards to their rights.

For those for whom religion is not a large part of their life, the removal of a religious exemption may not sound like a big deal. However, for those for whom religion makes up a center point for their lives the removal of a religious exemption is a critical thing. Many of the vaccines that are being mandated have been created on aborted fetal cells. Yes, aborted human fetus cells. This, for many people, would be an obvious religious concern, yet the right to make the choice based upon these convictions is being threatened or removed.

Another side to this coin is the potential of losing access to aspects of everyday life due to making the conscious choice to refuse vaccination. If the various exemptions are taken away, what you are actually taking away is the individual's right to then participate in society. What would be taken away? Let's begin with education. Currently, as previously mentioned, your child can still receive a public education without being fully vaccinated because there are legal exemptions for them to choose. When those exemptions are removed your child may then lose their right to a public education if they do not comply with the vaccination requirements. At the time of this writing, California and Louisiana have already made the new Covid vaccine mandatory for all children to be able to enter school. Now apply this concept to any business that wishes to make vaccines mandatory and not allow any exemptions and you can see how far reaching the effects could become. Think this is a far fetched idea? One need only to look at the current (Covid influenced) environment now to see how this is completely possible.

This is the reason why this topic is so incredibly important. If left to their own devices our government can and will take away all of our rights to make vaccine decisions. But wait, you say, our government would never do something like that. In 2018 the Argentinian government did exactly that…"Being vaccinated will be necessary and required for procedures such as entry and exit of the school system every year, processing or renewal of ID, passports, residence, medical procedures for work, prenuptial certificates, and driver's licenses, as well as for the processing of family allowances." You have no bodily choice if you are living in Argentina. If you think that this could only happen to them and not to us, think again. The District of Columbia recently passed the following Bill: "DC bill 23-171 states that "a minor, eleven years of age or older, may consent to receive a vaccine where the minor is capable of meeting the informed consent standard, and the vaccine is recommended by the United States Advisory Committee on Immunization Practices (ACIP)." But it doesn't stop there; the bill also prohibits the medical provider from documenting the vaccination in the medical record, restricting parents' ability to know the vaccination took place. (9) But this is only happening in DC, you say. Well, "A California lawmaker introduced a new bill that would allow children 12 and up to be vaccinated without parental consent. Right now, states like Alabama allow this at age 14, Oregon at 15, and Rhode Island and South Carolina at age 16. Only Washington, D.C. has a lower limit at age 11." (10) Those making the decisions want these vaccines in the arms of every single person and they do not care one bit about your right to bodily autonomy. Imagine your child legally getting a vaccine without your knowledge and no record of it happening. Now imagine your child having a severe reaction from this vaccine and you now have no knowledge as to what may be causing this reaction and therefore no ability to address this reaction properly. This sounds like a recipe for disaster to me.

This is why I decided to begin the book with this discussion. Our right to bodily autonomy, our right to make our own medical choices, should in no way be curtailed by our government. We should be in full control of what is done to us and to our children. It amazes me how ramped up I see people get when they are told that the government wants to take away their right to bear arms or their right to choose an abortion, however when told that the right to choose to be vaccinated or not is at risk, these same individuals think nothing of it. Regardless of whether or not you agree with anything else discussed in this book, this first point of health freedom/medical freedom should be the one point we can all agree upon. Take away this right and you are creating an incredibly slippery slope. Choosing what medical procedures are done to you or your child should be a fundamental right that no one should be able to usurp.

Point Number Two: History of Vaccines

"History will be kind to me for I intend to write it."
~ Winston Churchill

Perhaps you may have heard this particular quote, "History is written by the victors." There is much debate as to who said this, but the point still holds true. In 1492, Christopher Columbus sailed the ocean blue, and then what, he discovered America, correct? That is what thousands of young American kids were taught for generations. Turns out, not so true. Turns out he wasn't such a great guy either. Turns out he was at least partly responsible for the Atlantic slave trade and Native American genocide.(1) History with a twist. How about our lovely tradition of Thanksgiving? You know the one where a bunch of Native American Indians and settlers all sat down to enjoy a nice turkey dinner? Turns out they really did not like each other much, the fact was those Indians were most likely not even invited to this feast.(2) How about Paul Revere yelling, "The British are coming!" Or George Washington's wooden teeth? Even the date of the signing of the Constitution!(2) It most likely will surprise many, but history is not always what we may think it is.

If there is one point that has been brought up as an argument for the legitimacy of vaccines over and over again it is that history shows us that vaccines are incredibly successful and safe. This is the one comment I could always count on for someone to bring up at one of my seminars. I could show a hundred slides with every slide being research and documentation to illustrate that vaccines are not what we have been told they are and still there will be the one guy who stands up to ask the question I was waiting the entire seminar to have to answer, "What about polio?" It could as easily be, "What about measles?" Or even, "What about smallpox?" Whatever the given sickness, there is always someone who wants to tout the seemingly obvious success of past vaccines as having saved all of us from a life of misery, death and destruction. The thing is, is it really so obvious? Here is where things get interesting.

Probably the best book written on the subject of the history of vaccines is called Dissolving Illusions, by Suzanne Humphries, MD and Roman Bystrianyk. In this book the authors have done an excellent job of coordinating a mountainous amount of historical information in a manner that presents a clear and often disturbing view of the world during the 1800's and on up to our present time. The picture painted by the authors is not one that should be surprising to any one who reads it. It is a picture we are all familiar with simply through reading such classic books as Oliver Twist, A Tale of Two Cities or David CopperField. Read any of these books and they will give you a clear and often disturbing image of early life in America or Europe that shows the degrees of poverty and the unhygienic living conditions found especially within the larger cities. Life in large cities in America and Europe during the 1800's through to the early 1900's was not a particularly pretty picture. Living conditions were deplorable to say the least. The authors of Dissolving Illusions, give us a volume of quotes, photographs and documents illustrating the depth of problems such as sanitation, child labor, poor food supplies, the sorry state of the field of medicine and the overcrowding that occurred in big cities during that time period. One such quote from Dissolving Illusions that was particularly striking to me was this one regarding life in Chicago, "Before the 1870's, all kinds of garbage and human and animal waste had been thrown into what became known as the "North and South Sloughs"...(3, pg 10-11)" The quote goes on to explain that these "sloughs" drained sewage into the community's primary water source. This is but one small example of what life looked like in those early days. With overcrowding, poor food availability (or none), and human filth and waste running freely through the cities, is it any wonder that diseases were able to multiply, spread quickly, and kill large numbers of people?

The following is straight from the CDC's own website: "The 19th century shift in population from country to city that accompanied industrialization and immigration led to overcrowding in poor housing served by inadequate or nonexistent public water supplies and waste-disposal systems. These conditions resulted in repeated outbreaks of cholera, dysentery, tuberculosis (TB), typhoid fever, influenza, yellow fever, and malaria." They go on to say the following, "By 1900, however, the incidence of many of these diseases had begun to decline because of public health improvements, implementation of which continued into the 20th century. Local, state, and federal efforts to improve sanitation and hygiene reinforced the concept of collective "public health" action (e.g., to prevent infection by providing clean drinking water). By 1900, 40 of the 45 states had established health departments. The first county health departments were established in 1908. From the 1930s through the 1950s, state and local health departments made substantial progress in disease prevention activities, including sewage disposal, water treatment, food safety, organized solid waste disposal, and public education about hygienic practices (e.g., food-handling and hand-washing). Chlorination and other treatments of drinking water began in the early 1900s and became widespread public health practices, further decreasing the incidence of waterborne diseases. The incidence of TB also declined as improvements in housing reduced crowding and TB-control programs were initiated. In 1900, 194 of every 100,000 U.S. residents died from TB; most were residents of urban areas. In 1940 (before the introduction of antibiotic therapy), TB remained a leading cause of death, but the crude death rate had decreased to 46 per 100,000 persons."(4) So the CDC is saying that the incidence of TB was essentially .19% and without a vaccine it went down to an incidence of .05%.

"Animal and pest control also contributed to disease reduction. Nationally sponsored, state-coordinated vaccination and animal-control programs eliminated dog-to-dog transmission of rabies. Malaria, once endemic throughout the southeastern United States, was reduced to negligible levels by the late 1940s; regional mosquito-control programs played an important role in these efforts. Plague also diminished; the U.S. Marine Hospital Service (which later became the Public Health Service) led quarantine and ship inspection activities and rodent and vector-control operations. The last major rat-associated outbreak of plague in the United States occurred during 1924-1925 in Los Angeles. This outbreak included the last identified instance of human-to-human transmission of plague (through inhalation of infectious respiratory droplets from coughing patients) in this country."(4)

It is exactly this information regarding the dramatic drops in disease rates in conjunction with improvements to living conditions that seems to be spoken of out of one side of vaccine apologists mouths and then at the same time out of the other side of their mouths they say that it was the introduction of vaccines that saved mankind. Which was it? Either it was the vaccines that saved us or it was the change in living conditions that reduced the disease rates. Have you ever heard the expression, "you can't have your cake and eat it too?"

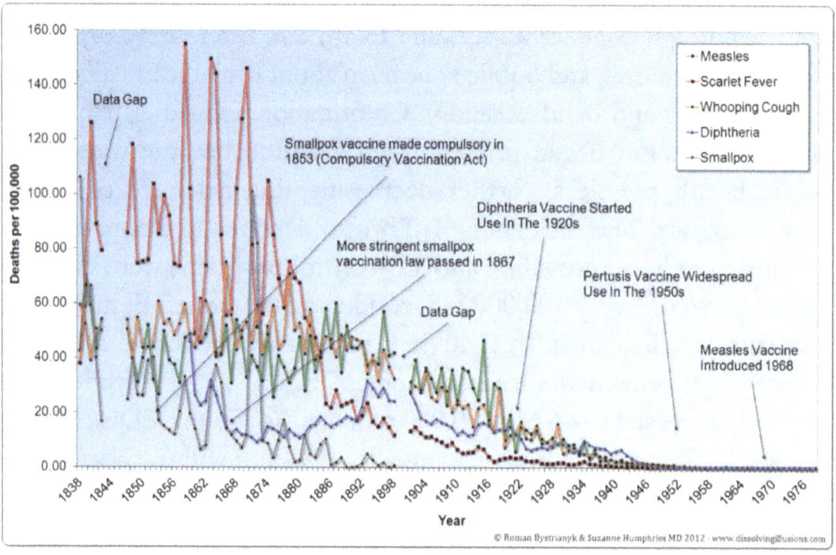

Graphs like the one shown above, taken from Dissolving Illusions, show a very different story to the cause of the drop in disease during the 1900's. These graphs were compiled utilizing information gathered from the CDC and other national archives. They clearly show disease rates dropping to all time lows well before the introduction vaccines. The authors of Dissolving Illusions had this to say about this apparent misuse of the information, "We are not saying that vaccines had absolutely no impact on deaths from these infectious diseases, but by using historical statistics, it is clear that most authors' claims regarding the lifesaving effect of vaccination are markedly exaggerated, and risk is continuously denied or underplayed. Despite the fact that "vaccines were responsible for the massive decline in deaths" is based on a false foundation, it permeates medical thinking all over the world." (3, pg. 473)

Look back at that graph and pay particular attention to Scarlet Fever. This was the scourge of the 1800's killing thousands of people. There has never been a vaccine created for Scarlet Fever, yet by the mid 1900's it had all but disappeared. Here's another one for you, the Black Death, or as it was also known as, the plague. During the 1300's, the Plague ran rampant over Europe. "Over the next five years, the Black Death would kill more than 20 million people in Europe—almost one-third of the continent's population." "The Black Death epidemic had run its course by the early 1350s, but the plague reappeared every few generations for centuries. Modern sanitation and public-health practices have greatly mitigated the impact of the disease but have not eliminated it. While antibiotics are available to treat the Black Death, according to The World Health Organization, there are still 1,000 to 3,000 cases of plague every year."(5) Here once again is another deadly disease that "went away" without a vaccine. A special mention to smallpox. Notice on the graph above that smallpox deaths had dropped incredibly from the early 1800's to the 1900's. Two things of note: first understand that even though the graph does refer to a "smallpox vaccine" as early as 1853, this "vaccine" was actually far more like a type of variolation (taking infected material directly from one source and transferring it to a non-infected person) than a vaccine. Because Jenner was taking infected material from cows (vacca) he termed the process vaccination. The process that was used in these earlier "vaccines" has no familiarity whatsoever with what we refer to as vaccines today. Secondly, not everyone agrees that it was inoculation (vaccination) that created the decrease in deaths. One paper titled The decline of adult smallpox in eighteenth-century London concluded that the dramatic drop in smallpox deaths "...shows little evidence of any impact of either inoculation or vaccination."(6)

A paper funded through Boston University and Harvard University titled The Questionable Contribution of Medical Measures to the Decline of Mortality in the United States in the Twentieth Century also strongly questioned the role that medical interventions (namely vaccines) had on the reduction of all sex mortality from 1900 to present. "In this paper we have attempted to dispel the myth that medical measures and the presence of medical services were primarily responsible for the modern decline in mortality." They went on to add that the change from medical intervention was "at most 3.5 percent of the total decline in mortality since 1900 could be ascribed to medical measures introduced for the diseases considered here."(7) This paper is chock full of wonderful graphs illustrating the drops in mortality prior to the introduction of vaccines.

Lastly, we are all told how vaccines saved us from measles. I hear this statement over and over again from vaccine proponents. Once again look at the graph above and notice that measles was well on the way out before the vaccine was introduced in 1963. "...deaths from measles in the United States decreased steadily throughout the 20th century—from approximately 12 per 100,000 population in 1912 to approximately 0.2 per 100,000 population in 1960."(11) Remember that the measles vaccine came out in 1963 and was not widespread until the 70's. The fact is that most of the big measles outbreaks over the past decades have been among heavily vaccinated populations. (7,8,9,10) The idea or belief that history proves that vaccines have been our saviors and prevented the devastation of mankind from a scourge of diseases is not the wonderful bedtime story that we have been told for so long. Did vaccines have an effect on various diseases over the past? To say that vaccines have had no effect on disease rates over time is likely false. However, glorifying the role of vaccines as the savior of mankind is more than false and sets up a perspective that places vaccines on a moral pedestal that can not be touched. That is exactly what has been created and that is what needs to be changed, otherwise we will continue down this same path where any mention of vaccines that is done in anything other than a devout voice is deemed blasphemous. As the old saying goes, Those that do not learn from history are doomed to repeat it. In this case, it is more a matter of learning the actual truth of our history so we do not continue lying to ourselves about vaccines.

Point Number Three: Media Bias and Censorship

"When propaganda is skillfully deployed, people are not even aware that their opinions are being manipulated."
~Noam Chomsky

Over the past decade, I have listened to news media and read magazine and newspaper articles regarding the topic of vaccines, and with extremely few exceptions, every last piece of news has covered the topic as though speaking from one voice. Media reporting on vaccines often demonstrates patterns of repetition and uniformity that suggests alignment with pharmaceutical industry narratives. Studies analyzing media coverage have shown that dissenting perspectives are underrepresented, which raises concerns about journalistic balance and the integrity of public discourse. Many of these facts that are being overlooked or ignored by those in the media are what make up the points that are being discussed in this book. I encourage you to look up every bit of referenced material on each of these points and then ask yourself the question, "If these references exist and can so easily be found, then why are they being so pointedly ignored by almost every media outlet and journalist? It is a very good question and one that everyone should consider when reading the information in these chapters.

One of my favorite things that is said over and over again is that the "science on vaccines is settled." If you were to type into a search engine the words "when is science settled," you will come up with a whole bunch of entries on a variety of topics and the one thing they all have in common will be the following, "Science is rarely, if ever, 'settled'. The nature of the scientific method – whereby hypotheses are routinely questioned, tested, refined and retested – is such that understanding is improved over time."(1) Those controlling the message continually say that vaccine science is settled and this gets picked up by all of the media and repeated over and over again as part of a script. This repetition seems to add even more credibility to the statement, even though the statement itself is false and no actual scientist would agree with any statement that professes that the science is ever settled. How does a journalist who has dedicated their life to the pursuit of truth buy into this ridiculous notion that science is ever settled? How do these same journalists forgo doing their own due diligence into a topic by not looking up the research for themselves? I can tell you how.

"It was calculated that in the first nine months of 2019, the pharmaceutical industry in the United States spent 4.54 billion U.S. dollars on direct-to-consumer (DTC) advertising. In the same period of 2018 the pharma sector spent 4.79 billion dollars, while the entire year spending amounted to 6.46 billion dollars."(2) In a paper written by a doctor of economics from Harvard the author stated, "The pharmaceutical industry would have you believe that advertising its products to the public is a good thing and, indeed, it is a very good thing—for the pharmaceutical industry. For every dollar spent on DTC advertising, the industry recoups $4.20. And last year it spent $4.22 billion. Just do the math to calculate the take-home bundle: more than the 2005 GDP of fifty countries, according to World Bank data. Add to that another $7.2 billion spent on direct-to-professional promotion in 2005, and it is no wonder that drug prices are higher here than anywhere else in the world"(3) Another article from the Center for Health Journalism had this to say regarding the pharmaceuticals influence on the media, "Local television news has, at times, been a cesspool of troubled advertising, sponsorship and content-sharing deals with vested interests in the healthcare industry. We've written about these issues more than 15 times but this is such a firmly-entrenched practice that we're not sure that another 15 articles would do any good."(4) How can anyone look at the financial influence that the pharmaceutical industry has in all of our media and say with any honesty that what we end up hearing and reading is the truth or simply that it is the truth that their sponsors wish us to hear? And it is.
getting worse.

We currently find ourselves living in a situation of Orwellian proportions. Sometime around March 2019, we began to see agencies demanding social media to move against anything that happened to question vaccine safety or effectiveness. The most surprising thing was the complicity of the social media companies. Pinterest has blocked searches for anti-vaccine information stating that this is spreading "misinformation." Amazon has taken down all "anti-vaccine" movies from their streaming service after receiving a letter from a State Representative. Facebook has "cracked" down on anything deemed "misinformation" about vaccines. Youtube has pulled all ads from videos with "anti-vaccine" content and has begun changing their algorithms to steer people away from "anti-vaccine" information. Youtube and Google's new algorithms will steer you towards pro vaccine information regardless of what you are searching for.(5) To make things even more interesting, there is a very obvious conflict of interest with Google which is moving quickly into the world of pharmaceuticals. "The company announced Tuesday strategic alliances with the pharmaceutical companies Novartis, Sanofi, Otsuka and Pfizer to help it move more deeply into the medical studies market. The goals for Verily (Google), and its pharma partners, are to reach patients in new ways, make it easier to enroll and participate in trials, and aggregate data across a variety of sources, including the electronic medical record or health-tracking wearable devices.(6)" And the news media covering all of this information has said not one word against this blatant censorship or the motives behind it. History is replete with examples of censorship by governments and regimes who forced their viewpoints and ideals on their citizens by burning books, taking over the media, controlling elections and persecution of its citizens. What is occurring with vaccines is no less than what we have seen throughout history. Yet, where is the outrage with what is going on today?

Meanwhile, the then (2019) head of the FDA, Scott Gottlieb, came out publicly and stated he thinks the U.S. government should step in and force mandatory vaccination on all children "Gottlieb told CNN that "certain states" could "force the hand of the federal health agencies" if they don't make changes." Changes meaning to eliminate all philosophical and religious exemptions from vaccines. In other words, take away all individual rights to what happens to their bodies! "Some states are engaging in such wide exemptions that they're creating the opportunity for outbreaks on a scale that is going to have national implications," the FDA head said in an interview with CNN.(7) The "outbreaks" Gottlieb is referring to were the "increased" cases of measles which occurred in 2019, these outbreaks had sparked panic among some people. Panic you say? For measles, you say? Yes, panic. Enough for the state of Washington to declare a statewide emergency because of 64 cases of measles. By the way folks, about 1 in 10,000 of measles cases are fatal. (8,9) That is a .01% chance of fatality. Back when I was growing up in the 1970's, measles was viewed as just another childhood illness that kids had to deal with. It was not looked at as a big deal. In fact, just to illustrate the point, there was an episode of the Brady Bunch from 1969 titled, "Is there a doctor in the house?" which revolved around all of the kids coming down with the measles at the same time. In this episode both of the parents and the two TV doctors that are brought to the house to look at the kids are all perfectly calm and look at the whole thing as no big deal. It was portrayed this way because that was exactly how people dealt with the measles back then. Now try to find this episode to watch on Hulu or Youtube or wherever. Good luck. It was easy to find until it started being used as the example I just gave and now it is being taken down and hidden so that it can not be used to illustrate a nonchalance about measles. In other words, it is being censored. And, by the way, the measles vaccine was not introduced until 1963 and was not even widespread in the U.S. until the 70's (meaning there was NO herd immunity effect in place at all). So, why suddenly is it worthy of a statewide emergency for 64 cases of a mostly non-fatal illness? I can not say for sure why, but how about to create hysteria? How about to create an atmosphere that will then tolerate the removal of freedom of speech and freedom of choice from medical tyranny? I did say Orwellian, did I not?

According to the First Amendment, "Congress shall make no law respecting an establishment of religion, or prohibiting the free exercise thereof; or abridging the freedom of speech, or of the press; or the right of the people peaceably to assemble, and to petition the Government for a redress of grievances." (10) This Amendment clearly states the freedom of speech and of religion. While the First Amendment may not apply to private companies like Facebook, it certainly does apply to our government getting involved and egging on these companies to censor information. How can any censorship of information meet this idea of freedom of speech? Also, how can the removal of an exemption to vaccines based on religion meet the idea of freedom of religion? The Fourth Amendment states, "The right of the people to be secure in their persons, houses, papers, and effects, against unreasonable searches and seizures, shall not be violated, and no Warrants shall issue, but upon probable cause, supported by Oath or affirmation, and particularly describing the place to be searched, and the persons or things to be seized." (10) If this Amendment is supposed to give people the "right to be secure in their persons," how can taking away my right to say no to injecting potentially deadly materials into my body or that of my child meet this idea? Last time I checked, these were rights granted to us as American citizens and protected by our Constitution. Last time I checked, we lived in a free and democratic country. How do any of the aforementioned acts meet what should be viewed as the standards of American freedoms? As a free and democratic nation, our right to free speech, religious freedom and to the sanctity of our bodies is a right that in no way should be allowed to be infringed upon.

As of this writing, we are seeing even more government intrusion into our civil liberties and encroachment into our constitutional rights. "The White House is asking social media companies to clamp down on chatter that deviates from officially distributed COVID-19 information as part of President Biden's "wartime effort" to vanquish the coronavirus. A senior administration official tells Reuters that the Biden administration is asking Facebook, Twitter and Google to help prevent anti-vaccine fears from going viral, as distrust of the inoculations emerges as a major barrier in the fight against the deadly virus."(11) This particular article goes on to say, "A Twitter spokesman said the company is "in regular communication with the White House on a number of critical issues including COVID-19 misinformation."

Firstly, the idea that the President can "vanquish" a virus is absurdity at its most high. But this whole idea of a variety of media companies bowing to the government to censor its users so that the government's message is not challenged is outrageous. Our government is "asking social media companies to clamp down on chatter that deviates from officially distributed COVID-19 information." How can we sit idly by and allow this to occur? Just the idea of our government asking to censor its citizens goes boldly in the face of everything our great nation is supposed to stand for. It is from the equal sharing of ideas that we learn and grow as humans and as a nation. When I, as an average citizen, can easily go online and find hundreds of research papers that support my findings about vaccines, then how can anyone say that this is misinformation? When only one idea or thought is allowed to be disseminated then the entire idea of freedom of speech, intelligent conversation and the furthering of scientific discourse and understanding are all stifled. For us as individuals to create an educated opinion and be able to make choices that greatly affect our lives and the lives of our loved ones, we must be able to read and view all sides of a topic. We must be able to utilize our intelligence to decide for ourselves what is truth and what is fiction. When our government steps in to tell us what we should or should not believe, or what we can and can not read or listen to; we are all in trouble.

According to Noam Chomsky, considered to be the father of modern linguistics, "propaganda is to democracy what the bludgeon is to a totalitarian state," and the mass media is the primary vehicle for delivering propaganda in the United States. Chomsky touches on how the modern public relations industry has been influenced by Walter Lippmann's theory of "spectator democracy," in which the public is seen as a "bewildered herd" that needs to be directed, not empowered; and how the public relations industry in the United States focuses on "controlling the public mind," and not on informing it.(12) I think that Mr. Chomsky has very accurately voiced our current environment in which we find ourselves.

More along the lines of "controlling the public mind" becomes clear when you look at this information that came from an article written in Scientific American regarding control of the media. "Documents obtained by Scientific American through Freedom of Information Act requests now paint a disturbing picture of the tactics that are used to control the science press. For example, the FDA assures the public that it is committed to transparency, but the documents show that, privately, the agency denies many reporters access—including ones from major outlets such as Fox News—and even deceives them with half-truths to handicap them in their pursuit of a story. At the same time, the FDA cultivates a coterie of journalists whom it keeps in line with threats. The agency has made it a practice to demand total control over whom reporters can and can't talk to until after the news has broken, deaf to protests by journalistic associations and media ethicists and in violation of its own written policies. A document from January 2014, describes the FDA's strategy for getting media coverage of the launch of a new public health ad campaign. It lays out a plan for the agency to host a "media briefing for select, top-tier reporters who will have a major influence on coverage and public opinion of the campaigns.... Media who attend the briefing will be instructed that there is a strict, close-hold embargo that does not allow for contact with those outside of the FDA for comment on the campaign." "The media briefing will give us an opportunity to shape the news stories, conduct embargoed interviews with the major outlets ahead of the launch and give media outlets opportunities to prepare more in-depth coverage of the campaign launch." One reporter commented, "In that situation, the journalist is allowing his or her reporting hands to be tied in a way that they're not going to be anything, ultimately, other than a stenographer." The author of the article went on noting that it "will be a serious obstacle to good journalism. Reporters who want to be competitive on a story will essentially have to agree to write only what the FDA wants to tell the world, without analysis or outside commentary."(13)

Ask yourself why you have not read or heard anything that you will find in this book debated or discussed in the newspapers you read or the news programs you watch. Why, when you read articles regarding vaccines or watch news programs about vaccines do you only hear that vaccines are great and that anyone who says otherwise is an "anti-vaxxer?" In fact, if the news media says anything about someone who is bringing up points against vaccines they are spoken of as bad, ridiculous, crazy or harmful. Never do they stop for even one second and say, "maybe we should look into this or have a conversation about it." If you speak out against vaccines you are risking your reputation and possibly your livelihood. (14,15,16,17,18,19,20) Even legendary musician Eric Clapton, who released a video telling people that he felt he had a reaction to the Covid vaccine, was not immune from the harsh criticism. (21) The only thing he was guilty of was sharing his negative vaccine experience. He did not say all vaccines were bad, nor did he tell everyone not to get the vaccine. He simply shared his experience and for doing this has had a world of grief over doing so. Actress Evangeline Lilly went to the Defeat the Mandates March on Washington (January 23, 2022) and said that "I was in DC this weekend to support bodily sovereignty." For that she was blasted by the media for being an "anti-vaxxer" and for spreading "misinformation." (22,23) If you are against vaccines, if you even question vaccines, you are seen as against humanity. Far too many people fail to see this and catch the insanity and the blatantly obvious problem with this situation. Shouldn't we want to know the truth? Shouldn't we be demanding that our media show a balanced viewpoint and not kowtow to the pharmaceutical industry and to our government? As Jim Morrison once said, "Whoever controls the media, controls the mind."

Point Number Four: Trust for a Liability Free Product

"It is wrong and immoral to seek to escape the consequences of one's acts."
~Mahatma Gandhi

Let me ask you a couple of serious questions. I want you to truly think about your answer before giving it. If you were going to purchase a vehicle for your young teen who was just beginning to drive, which vehicle would you be more likely to purchase? Vehicle one is manufactured by a company that is fully liable for any and all manufacturing defects that may occur to said vehicle. Vehicle two is manufactured by a company who has been given a pass for all liability. This second company has zero responsibility for any injuries or deaths that may occur to your teenager while driving the vehicle that they have created. Which vehicle are you going to purchase for your teen? Next question. You need to purchase medication to help your child to be able to live with a particular condition. Medication number one is created by a pharmaceutical company that is held liable for any problems that may occur to your child from taking their product. Medication number two is created by a pharmaceutical company that has been given a complete pass for any and all liability from any and all injuries or death that may occur to your child while taking their product. Which medication will you be purchasing for your child? Did it take you long to answer these questions? Most likely these were easy choices for you. So how do questions like these have anything to do with vaccines?

In 1986, in response to an onslaught of lawsuits against vaccine manufacturers for vaccine related injuries, pharmaceutical companies threatened Congress that they would stop manufacturing vaccines unless they had protection from liability. Congress caved to this pressure and passed the National Vaccine Injury Act (NVIA) and its partner the National Vaccine Injury Compensation Program (NVICP). These two programs were set up to relieve vaccine manufacturers of all liability for injury or death related to the vaccine products that they create. "The National Vaccine Injury Compensation Program is a no-fault alternative to the traditional legal system for resolving vaccine injury petitions. The reasoning, from the pharmaceutical companies perspective, was that lawsuits against vaccine companies and health care providers threatened to cause vaccine shortages and reduce U.S. vaccination rates, which could have caused a resurgence of vaccine preventable diseases."(1) Great idea, right? The U.S. government, in response to the vaccine manufacturers threatening them with a stop in production of vaccines, allowed them to continue making their products but now with zero liability. Genius. Instead, through the NVICP the government would, supposedly, take on the liability aspect of vaccines.

This new program (NVIC) was supposedly a great alternative. The pharmaceutical companies continue to make the vaccines, while the government takes care of any liability for their product. Win-win right? The problems (which should have been evident from the start) however are multiple. First, giving any corporation carte blanche to do whatever they wish to do is incredibly naive and short sighted. Secondly, you are now placing the responsibility to litigate these cases into the hands of our government which does not have the best track record at making situations easy or fluid. The problems with this system began almost immediately and continue up to this day. One issue has been the length of time it takes to go through litigation, "VICP claims filed since fiscal year 1999 took an average of about 5 and a half years to adjudicate, according to U.S. Court of Federal Claims data for the nearly 8,800 claims filed since fiscal year 1999..."(3) You could make the argument that all court cases can take a long time to come to closure, however you would (and should) expect that when our government decided to take over the responsibility for these cases involving families with children who died or were injured by mandated vaccines, that the cases would be handled in a more timely fashion. Even more, in a 2014 report by the US Government Accountability Office to the Chairman, Committee on Oversight and Government Reform,

House of Representatives the reviews by individuals who had used this service had these statements to say:

- "view the vaccine injury claims process as confusing, time-consuming, too lengthy, and traumatic"

- "to the question on the amount of compensation reported the award amount was inadequate to cover past and future medical care."

- "the perception of an adversarial or unfriendly environment throughout the process, the use of settlements and perceived pressure to settle claims"

- "HRSA noted that one of the critical issues facing the program from 2005 to 2010 was that many parents, the general public, attorneys, and health care professionals were not aware VICP existed."

- "One stakeholder commented that the public is largely unaware of the program, and this lack of awareness contributes to missing filing deadlines and individuals being denied the opportunity for compensation" (3)

Add to this the incredible difficulty in getting a medical doctor to actually sign off that you or your child was actually injured by a vaccine (which is necessary to even get this process started). In a special report delivered to The Agency for Healthcare Research and Quality (AHRQ) U.S. Department of Health and Human Services, it was reported that less than 1% of vaccine injuries are ever reported.(4)

As for giving a pharmaceutical company carte blanche to make a product for the masses, this is where it becomes confusing that anyone would have allowed this arrangement to be created in the first place. Just check out these lawsuits (the ones that I could easily find by the way) that have been settled against the various big pharmaceutical companies. I would apologize for this list being so long but you really would need to blame the pharma companies and not me for that.

- "Pharmaceutical giant Purdue Pharma LP secretly pursued a plan, dubbed "Project Tango," to become "an end-to-end pain provider" by selling both opioids and drugs to treat opioid addiction, all while owners on the board – members of one of America's richest families – reaped more than $4 billion in opioid profits." "In 2001, the lawsuit says, Sackler in a confidential email disclosed "his solution to the overwhelming evidence of overdose and death: blame and stigmatize people who become addicted to opioids."(5)

- "American pharmaceutical company Merck, Sharp & Dohme was sentenced by U.S. District Court Judge Patti B. Saris in Boston to pay a criminal fine in the amount of $321,636,000 in connection with its guilty plea related to its promotion and marketing of the painkiller Vioxx (Rofecoxib), the Justice Department announced today. In December 2011, Merck pleaded guilty to violating the Food, Drug and Cosmetic Act (FDCA) for introducing a misbranded drug, Vioxx, into interstate commerce."(6) "Research published in the medical journal *Lancet* estimates that 88,000 Americans had heart attacks from taking Vioxx, and 38,000 of them died."(7)

- "Merck made a "hit list" of doctors who criticized Vioxx, according to testimony in a Vioxx class action case in Australia. The list, emailed between Merck employees, contained doctors' names with the labels "neutralize," "neutralized" or "discredit" next to them."(8)

- "Amgen accepted $612m as civil liability and $150m as criminal fine and forfeiture in 2007 for illegally introducing Aranesp into interstate commerce."(9)

- "Bayer and J & J jointly resolved approximately 25,000 claims filed in the US federal and state courts against their anticoagulant drug, Xarelto, in 2019. The lawsuits alleged that the two companies downplayed the risks related to Xarelto and marketed the drug as a substitute to another anticoagulant, warfarin, to avoid fatal blood clots."(9)

- "TAP Pharmaceuticals paid approximately $875m for fraudulent drug pricing and marketing practices for its prostate cancer drug, Lupron. The settlement amount included $290m as a criminal fine, $559.4m for filing false and misleading claims with the Medicare and Medicaid programmes, as well as $25.5m for filing false and misleading claims."(9)

- "Eli Lilly paid a $515m criminal fine and up to $800m as civil settlements to resolve allegations related to the unlawful promotion of its antipsychotic drug Zyprexa in 2009."(9)

- "In 2012, Abbott Laboratories pleaded guilty to unlawfully promoting its prescription drug Depakote, which resulted in a $700m criminal fine and forfeiture, in addition to $800m in civil settlements."(9)

- "Johnson & Johnson paid a $485m as a criminal fine and forfeiture and $1.72bn as civil settlements to settle various misconduct charges filed in 2013."(9)

- "Pfizer and its subsidiary Pharmacia & Upjohn Company paid $2.3bn to settle criminal and civil liabilities for illegal promotion of their pharmaceutical products."(9)

- J&J to Pay $70 Million to Settle Cases Brought by SEC and Criminal Authorities "J&J chose profit margins over compliance with the law by acquiring a private company for the purpose of paying bribes, and using sham contracts, off-shore companies, and slush funds to cover its tracks."(13)

- "Takeda Pharmaceutical settled approximately 8,000 federal and state lawsuits over its oral diabetes drug Actos (pioglitazone) by paying $2.4bn in 2015. The company was found guilty of hiding the bladder cancer risks related to the drug."(9)

- "GlaxoSmithKline (GSK) settled the biggest ever healthcare lawsuit in history with a $3bn payment in 2012. The company pleaded guilty to three counts and paid $1bn as a criminal penalty and $2bn to resolve civil liabilities. GSK was found guilty of unlawfully promoting certain prescription drugs such as Paxil, Wellbutrin, and Avandia. It failed to report certain safety data to the FDA and reported false drug prices to underpay rebates owed under the Medicaid Drug Rebate Program."(9)

- "Actelion Pharmaceuticals used a foundation to illegally pay copays for thousands of Medicare patients taking [their] drugs, which would also induce patients to buy them because the prices would be higher otherwise. It essentially set up a fund to cover copays of its own drugs, which undermines the Medicare copay structure which is designed to prevent drug price inflation. Actelion was then able to raise the price of Tracleer by nearly 30 times the overall rate of inflation."(10)

- "AstraZeneca Pharmaceutical was marketing the drug (Seroquel) for additional uses...even though the FDA hadn't approved Seroquel for those uses. In addition, AstraZeneca paid kickbacks to doctors for authoring articles about the drug being used in ways that weren't approved."(10)

- "Abbott Laboratories promoted Depakote as a drug to control agitation and aggression in elderly dementia patients, and for schizophrenia. The FDA hadn't approved the drug for either of these uses. For 8 years, the manufacturer marketed Depakote for this purpose in nursing homes, even though there wasn't any evidence that the drug was safe and effective when used that way. Criminal fines in this action were $700 million and civil settlements were $800 million."(10)

Ongoing lawsuits:

- ZH Pharmaceuticals: "People who took the blood pressure drug Valsartan and were diagnosed with cancer are suing the companies that made and distributed the tainted medications. The lawsuits allege that Valsartan batches were contaminated with NDMA, a potential carcinogen."(11)

- "Zostavazx is a vaccine used to prevent shingles. This class action claim is against Merck, a drug manufacturer that failed to warn doctors and patients that this vaccine can cause shingles."(11)

- "Tenofovir is a prescription medication used to treat HIV and hepatitis B infections. This medication led to kidney disease and bone injuries in some patients. Gilead Sciences, the manufacturer, was aware of the risk but never removed it from the market."(11)

- "Pradaxa is a blood thinner that treats blood clots and prevents stroke. This prescription drug was unfortunately linked to an overwhelming number of severe bleeding cases, including several fatalities. There have been many wrongful death lawsuits filed against drug manufacturer Boehringer Ingelheim because of Pradaxa."(11)

- "Viberzi (made by Allergan Pharmaceutical) treats diarrhea and abdominal pain for irritable bowel syndrome (IBS). The lawsuit stems from a failure to warn patients and doctors that people missing their gallbladder are at risk of pancreatitis. The FDA was made aware of over 100 reports of patients who contracted pancreatitis as a result of Viberzi."(11)

- "Jardiance helps lower blood sugar in patients with type 2 diabetes. This prescription drug, along with Farixga, can increase the risk of contracting Fournier's Gangrene. The lawsuits claim that the drug manufacturer (Boehringer Ingelheim and Eli Lilly and Company) failed to warn patients about this risk."(11)

- "Zantac is a medication designed to treat and prevent heartburn. It may also treat gastroesophageal reflux disease (GERD) and stomach ulcers. Zantac was reported to be contaminated with a substance that causes cancer. The lawsuit alleges drug makers Sanofi and Boehringer Ingelheim should have known about this cancer-causing chemical."(11)

- "These over-the-counter medications, Nexium (AstraZeneca) and Prilosec (Proctor and Gamble) treat heartburn, stomach ulcers, and GERD. Thousands of lawsuits have been filed against the manufacturer by people who have suffered stroke, bone fractures, heart damage, and other injuries as a result of long-term use."(11)

- "Antidepressants are another type of prescription drug involved in class action lawsuits. Some reported side effects of antidepressants include increased suicidal ideation and behavior in adults, teens, and children." Prozac-Eli Lilly & Co., Paxil-Apotex Corp., Zoloft-Pfizer, Lexapro-Forest Laboratories Inc."(11)

- Hoffmann-La Roche bilked U.S. federal and state governments out of $1.5 billion by misrepresenting clinical studies and falsely claiming that its well-known influenza medicine Tamiflu was effective at containing potential pandemics. (12)

And this is not even a complete list!

Trust is a funny thing. I have heard that expression before, however I am not so sure I really agree or understand it. Is trust a funny thing? It should be a pretty straightforward thing. A person, or in this example a corporation, creates trust through their actions. Show me you can be trustworthy and the trust comes as a byproduct of your actions. All of the above legal actions against the various pharmaceutical companies all have occurred or are occurring while these companies were being held accountable for their actions. These companies all had liability for their actions and still ended up in their individual legal entanglements. Most of these companies repeated their illegal actions over and over again. If the mountain of lawsuits does not sway you, add one more ingredient to this noxious soup, the Vaccines Market will be worth $58.4 billion by 2024. (13) Money, especially when it reaches amounts such as this, motivates corporations to do all sorts of things. Unfortunately, these are usually not the humanitarian sort of things. Should I perhaps bring up the tobacco industry and how it was shown that they knew all the bad things about their product for decades and did nothing at all to stop what they were doing? Maybe the pharmaceutical companies are totally different from the tobacco industry. Perhaps they care nothing about affecting their profits. Or maybe I should bring up the ongoing lawsuits against the 3M Company, the Chemours Company and DuPont who are all being charged with knowingly releasing hazardous chemicals into the environment? "Lori Swanson, the former Minnesota attorney general who sued 3M for contamination of her state, said the company "knew about the risks of the chemicals to the drinking water, the environment and human health for decades but concealed its knowledge, subverted the science and kept pushing the chemicals out the door." (14)

The most incredibly bizarre thing is that people, even after knowing all of this information, will still fight tooth-and-nail arguing about how safe and effective vaccines are. I wonder if they realize that the vast majority of research regarding these vaccines was bought and paid for by the very same companies that created these no liability products? (15) You have a product made by companies that have zero liability for said product. Companies that have a long history of knowingly lying and harming the public with their products. And these same companies have financial ties to the bureaucracy that is supposed to regulate these products.(16)(17) Perhaps you can read about all of this and still trust that these companies have your best interests in mind when they create the vaccines for you and your children. Or perhaps you can see through the layers of lies and deceit and understand that their motivations may not be quite so pure. At the very least, this information should begin to raise some doubts.

Point Number Five
Conflicts of interest

"Today everything is a conflict of interest."
~ Sid Vicious

The idea of conflicts of interest is an incredibly convoluted topic when it comes to vaccines, as there are conflicts coming from a multitude of sources and directions. Conflicts abound in the FDA, the CDC, the pharmaceutical companies themselves, the medical journals, and in the legislative bodies. It is no small wonder why so many individuals are questioning the motives behind the entire vaccine industry. With so many people distorting the truth (or outright lying) it is easy to begin believing that something nefarious is at hand. Let's explore some of these conflicts and you can make up your own opinion after seeing even a (very) small sampling of what can be found out there.

Conflicts in Medical Journals

Giovanni Fava, MD, is a professor of psychiatry at both the University of Bologna and the University of Buffalo School of Medicine and Biomedical Sciences and has written extensively on the subject of explicit bias within the field of psychiatry, specifically within the medical journals. The following is taken from a paper he wrote titled "Financial conflicts of interest in psychiatry," "Scientific societies may control medical journals and affect editorial policies and the selection of papers. Further, financial ties may also affect the scientific meetings of those societies. This is something anyone walking in a major society meeting may easily perceive." "It has been repeatedly reported that studies sponsored by pharmaceutical companies are more likely to have outcomes favorable to the sponsor. Industry sponsorship also results in restrictions on publication and data sharing and in selective reporting. Perlis et al. examined funding sources and authors' financial conflicts of interest in clinical trials published in four leading American journals concerned with psychiatry. Sixty percent were funded by a pharmaceutical industry, and conflict of interest was associated with a greater likelihood of reporting a drug to be superior to placebo. Further, Melander et al. analyzed controlled studies of selective serotonin reuptake inhibitors and found that sponsored studies with favorable results were more often published than negative studies. A good example of this selective publication is given by the scandal following the finding that a major pharmaceutical company allegedly withheld from the medical community clinical trial findings which indicated that a widely used antidepressant had no beneficial effect in treating adolescents. This casts serious doubt on the representativeness of the drug trials which are included in meta analysis. Further, even systematic reviews require careful critical appraisal. Conflicts of interest may affect this appraisal. Evidence-based medicine may thus be a deceptive instrument of propaganda." Even though Dr. Fava specializes in looking at the field of psychiatry he went on to make this comment, "The problem of conflicts of interest in psychiatry does not appear to be different from other fields of clinical medicine." He went even further in this paper to imply even deeper conflicts of interest within his industry by saying there was, "growing concern about the relationship between the World Health Organization (WHO) and the pharmaceutical industry." (1)

The idea of problems within the world of medical journals is not a new issue nor is it limited to any one field. In another article titled "Pharmaceutical advertising revenue and physician organizations: how much is too much?," the authors concluded that "Potential financial conflicts of interest arising from pharmaceutical advertisements in medical journals may be substantial." (2) Besides bias coming from obvious financial conflicts of interest, the bias can come from the way(s) in which a study is actually published. In the article, "Evidence b(i)ased medicine--selective reporting from studies sponsored by pharmaceutical industry: review of studies in new drug applications, the authors found that "The degree of multiple publication, selective publication, and selective reporting differed between products. Thus, any attempt to recommend a specific selective serotonin reuptake inhibitor from the publicly available data only is likely to be based on biased evidence." (3) This study was regarding SSRI's not vaccines, however it is an issue that affects all study publications. This "publication bias" seems to be everywhere and influences what and how studies are sometimes published such as burying negative results, "it appears that the literature is predominantly biased toward positive results, of which many are likely to be false, whereas negative results that are more likely to be true negative results are disappearing." (4) Another article had this to say, "The evidence is strong that companies are getting the results they want, and this is especially worrisome because between two-thirds and three-quarters of the trials published in the major journals are funded by the industry." "The companies seem to get the results they want not by fiddling the results, which would be far too crude and possibly detectable by peer review, but rather by asking the "right" questions—and there are many ways to do this. ...there are many ways to hugely increase the chance of producing favorable results, and there are many hired guns who will think up new ways and stay one jump ahead of peer reviewers." (5)

Unfortunately, if a pharmaceutical company wants a positive study result there are ways they can help to ensure that it occurs. "In a desire to find a positive outcome of the study, authors can succumb to the pitfalls of focusing on the positive rather than the negative. Facing non-significant results authors can decide to tweak the hypothesis to better suit their data, also known as HARKing (hypothesizing after the results are known). HARKing entails meticulous examination or complete disregard of the data that does not fit into the tested hypothesis. In addition, there are numerous reports of scientific misconduct where scientists have completely falsified the published data." (6) In fact, "according to a survey published in the journal *Nature* last summer, more than 70% of researchers have tried and failed to reproduce another scientist's experiments." (7) All of this should leave you wondering if you can trust what the pharmaceutical companies want us to believe. You will see this exact example of "HARKing" in the Point concerning autism.

In an eye opening article by journalist Martha Rosenberg, she revealed the top five ways big pharma influences doctors. One of the top five was "ghost writing" for medical journals. "Being published in medical journals is essential to academic doctors but researching, writing and reworking papers is a formidable job. Luckily for doctors, Pharma is willing to help—as long as they write what Pharma wants. In just three years, medical writers associated with Parke-Davis, which became Pfizer, wrote 13 papers extolling the benefits of Neurontin, including in the prestigious Cleveland Clinic Journal of Medicine, in the names of the "author" doctors. Medical writers at Wyeth, also now Pfizer, wrote more than 50 papers pushing the controversial Hormone Replacement Therapy (HRT) in the names of doctor "authors." Another of her top five is "speakers bureaus." "Despite academic restrictions, faculty at many top institutions including division chiefs "stay on the industry lecture circuit, where they can net tens of thousands in additional income," reported ProPublica in 2010. Even at the prestigious Cleveland Clinic where the chairman of cardiovascular medicine, Steven E. Nissen, calls industry-paid speakers "whores," the practice flourishes, ProPublica reported." She also lists clinical trials as part of her top five. "Not all clinical trials are kosher. Another sneaky way Pharma gets doctors to prescribe its drugs is to set up faux clinical trials to influence doctors. A 1995 study billed as assessing the safety, efficacy and tolerability of Neurontin was nothing but a ruse to get the 772 participating doctors to prescribe the drug, said an article in the Archives of Internal Medicine, because it gave them familiarity and experience with the drug. (This indirect sales job parallels what is said to happen with speaker's bureaus: the speakers may not convince anyone else, but they begin prescribing the drug themselves.) In addition to misleading the doctors who thought the trials were valid, the study also misled the patients who did not know it was a marketing, or "seeding" study, and whose participation was overseen by investigators with insufficient training and clinical experience. Eleven of the 2,759 patients in the trials died, 73 suffered severe adverse events and 997 experienced less serious side-effects."(8)

Conflicts in the FDA

The following is from an article posted in USA Today, September 25, 2000: "More than half of the experts hired to advise the government on the safety and effectiveness of medicine have financial relationships with the pharmaceutical companies that will be helped or hurt by their decisions, a [USA TODAY] study found. These experts are hired to advise the Food and Drug Administration on which medicines should be approved for sale, what the warning labels should say and how studies of drugs should be designed. The experts are supposed to be independent, but USA TODAY found that 54% of the time they have a direct financial interest in the drug or topic they are asked to evaluate. These conflicts include helping a pharmaceutical company develop a medicine, then serving on an FDA advisory committee that judges the drug. Federal law generally prohibits the FDA from using experts with financial conflicts of interest, but the FDA has waived the restriction more than 800 times since 1998." (9) A separate article, this one from *Science* Magazine titled "Hidden conflicts? Pharma payments to FDA advisers after drug approvals spark ethical concerns," said similar things regarding the FDA..."fits a pattern of what might be called pay-later conflicts of interest, which have gone largely unnoticed—and entirely unpoliced. In examining compensation records from drug companies to physicians who advised FDA on whether to approve 28 psychopharmacologic, arthritis, and cardiac or renal drugs between 2008 and 2014, *Science* found widespread after-the-fact payments or research support to panel members. The agency's safeguards against potential conflicts of interest are not designed to prevent such future financial ties. Other apparent conflicts may have also slipped by: Science found that at the time of or in the year leading up to the advisory meetings, many of those panel members...received payments or other financial support from the drugmaker or key competitors for consulting, travel, lectures, or research. FDA did not publicly note those financial ties." (10) This article, titled "Conflicts of Interest are Common at FDA," repeated this same idea, "In 73% of the 221 meetings analyzed, at least one advisory member or consultant had one or more conflicts." "In at least 32 cases, patient advocacy groups that were funded by a drug company provided speakers during the public sessions, and in 47 instances a public speaker was flown in by a drug sponsor. This, said the researchers, "amplifies the growing concern that pharmaceutical industry sponsorship is becoming more prominent in nonprofit, patient advocacy groups that were once viewed as grassroots organizations independent of industry influence." (11) "Big Pharma is also the biggest defrauder of the Federal Government under the False Claims Act, according to consumer watchdog group Public Citizen. Big Pharma contributes heavily to the annual budget of the U.S. Food and Drug Administration. Big Pharma does this through application fees (user fees) for its new products. Experts say the industry contributes about two thirds of the FDA's budget. Big Pharma also uses its profits and an army of 1,378 paid lobbyists to spread its influence on Capitol Hill." (12)

Conflicts within the Legislative Bodies

When you begin to understand the vast amount of dollars funneled into lobbying by the pharmaceutical industry you can begin to understand the influence they create on all governmental bodies. The money the pharmaceutical companies spend each year is staggering. "Pharmaceutical and health product industry spending on federal lobbying averaged $233 million per year. Contributions were targeted at senior legislators in Congress involved in drafting health care laws and state committees that opposed or supported key referenda on drug pricing and regulation." (13) One article had this to say regarding the financial influence, "Why, when confronted with policy alternatives that could improve patient care, public health, and the economy, does Congress neglect those goals and tailor legislation to suit the interests of pharmaceutical corporations? In brief, for generations, the pharmaceutical industry has convinced legislators to define policy problems in ways that protect its profit margin. It reinforces this framework by selectively providing information and by targeting campaign contributions to influential legislators and allies." (14) To see how the pharmaceutical industry uses this enormous financial budget to push their agendas regardless of morals and ethics one needs look no further than the recent opioid crisis. The Associated Press printed an article in 2016 titled "Pharma lobbying held deep influence over policies on on opioids." In this article the authors "analyzed data on how the companies and their allies deployed lobbyists and contributed to political campaigns." Their findings showed that the drug companies had specific branches of lobbyists dedicated to opioids and that the "opioid lobby's political spending adds up to more than eight times what the formidable gun lobby recorded for political activities during the same period." (15) The article goes on to illustrate a myriad of ways in which the opioid lobby worked to help increase their specific industry. Remember that the pharmaceutical industry is in this for themselves. This is not about selfless service to others. In an article titled "FDA medical adviser: 'Congress is Owned by Pharma,' " it discussed the quagmire of corruption and potential corruption that surrounds this industry. In the article Dr. Raeford Brown, a pediatric anesthesia specialist at the UK Kentucky Children's Hospital and chair of the Food and Drug Administration (FDA) Committee on Analgesics and Anesthetics is quoted, "I'm really much more concerned because Congress is supposed to have oversight for the FDA," Brown said. "If the FDA isn't going to hold pharma accountable, and Congress is getting paid to not hold pharma accountable, then it really doesn't matter who the president is because it's really about Congress." The article goes into detail regarding the amount of money that the pharmaceutical industry pours into congress. To see the vast amount of money talked about for yourself, you can go to opensecrets.org, a website operated by the nonpartisan Center for Responsive Politics, which tracks money in U.S. politics. (16) In yet another issue involving congress, the Roosevelt Institute produced a brief called "Capturing the Government: Big Pharma's Take Over of Policymaking" where they concluded that "The capture of our government by the pharmaceutical industry has societal consequences beyond drug price and health safety." (17) One of the influences that they pointed out was the "revolving door between government service and pharmaceutical industry positions."

Conflict of revolving doors

The revolving door generally refers to 'an institutionalized system or culture of integration between government officials and regulated economic interests.' When individuals 'revolve' back and forth between regulatory agencies and the firms they regulate, it can create both actual and perceived perverse incentive structures and conflicts of interest." (18) "Seven Democratic U.S. senators on Thursday introduced legislation designed to slow the 'revolving door' between federal agencies such as the Drug Enforcement Administration and the pharmaceutical companies they regulate. It is not unusual for corporations to hire federal employees directly from the government, nor for industry officials to join the government in high-ranking positions. There are regulations designed to prevent potential conflicts of interest. Government ethics experts say some of those laws are easily skirted." (19) The system of the revolving door between government and the pharmaceutical industry has been an issue for a very long time with nothing being done regarding it. The following is a small sampling of this revolving door:

- "Commissioner Scott Gottlieb is just the latest administration official to go through the revolving door after his second tour at the FDA. Gottlieb recently resigned from his spot as the top federal drug regulator to take on a role at Pfizer—the top drug producer in the United States. The move came with a nice cash bonus as well, as stock options doubled the former commissioner's income to upwards of $330,000. In his time as head of the FDA, Gottlieb lowered the number of inspections at both foreign and domestic drug manufacturers producing drugs sold in the United States. He also sped up the approval process for experimental and generic drugs, leading many to question whether the 'newer and cheaper' drugs hitting the market were actually safe. Those policies directly benefited Big Pharma bottom lines." (20)

- "Michael R. Taylor, a lawyer for Monsanto for several years became deputy commissioner for policy at the Food and Drug Administration (FDA) and then Administrator of the Food Safety & Inspection Service of the Dept of Agriculture. He afterwards became Monsanto's Vice President for Public Policy and then senior fellow at the think tank Resources for the Future. In 2010 he was appointed deputy commissioner for foods at the FDA." (21)

- "Current Health and Human Services Secretary Alex Azar—Gottlieb's former boss—used to be president of Lilly USA, the U.S. branch of pharmaceutical giant Eli Lilly." (20)

- "Julie L. Gerberding left her position as the head of the CDC and became the President of Merk's vaccine division. She has a current personal net worth of 15.2 million dollars." (22)

- "Like John Stone, Ryan Long and Brent Del Monte, many ex-Hill staffers working in some way for the pharmaceutical industry came from key committees, including the Senate Committee on Health, Education, Labor and Pensions (HELP) and the House Energy and Commerce Committee." (23)

In another study by the Roosevelt Institute they stated that "an active and sizable revolving door exists between the pharmaceutical industry and government, creating opportunities to influence the policymaking of FDA regulators, congressional staffers, and agency heads. The revolving door extends to the halls of Congress, as well. A 2018 analysis from Kaiser Health News found nearly 340 former congressional staffers work for drug companies or their lobbying firms, many from key committees, and that dozens of former employees of drug companies worked as congressional staffers as of January 2018. An investigation from the Sunlight Foundation found the average chief of staff increases their salary by 40 percent when they move to the private sector." (24) They went on in this article to state, "The undue influence the pharmaceutical industry exerts over government officials is so pervasive and commonplace that many accounts of corruption fail to describe its real-world consequences. When we broaden our view of corruption to include the common yet deeply troubling influence the pharmaceutical industry exerts over nearly every part of our regulatory and policymaking apparatus, it becomes clear that industry capture has consequences for patients, public health, and the broader social welfare." (24) Two researchers from Oregon Health and Science University "tracked 55 FDA reviewers in the hematology-oncology field from 2001 through 2010, using LinkedIn, PubMed and other publicly available job data. The researchers found that of the 26 reviewers who left the FDA during this period, 15 of them, or 57 percent, later worked or consulted for the biopharmaceutical industry. Put another way, about 27 percent of the total number of reviewers left their federal oversight posts to work for the industry they previously regulated."(25) This revolving door process continues unchecked today.

Conflicts with the CDC

If an individual owned a patent for a product and was subsequently placed in a position of power over what occurs with that same product, would you not think that is a conflict of interest? I certainly would. "Each of the 12 members of the CDC's ACIP (Advisory Committee on Immunization Practices) has a significant influence on the health of nearly every individual of the American population. Because they are responsible for adding to and/or altering the national vaccine schedule, it is of critical importance that they remain objective and unbiased before determining whether a new vaccination is appropriate for use, particularly in the bodies of vulnerable young children. Unfortunately, a significant number of ACIP members receive direct financial returns when more vaccinations are added to the current schedule. Many own vaccination related patent(s) and/or stock shares of the pharmaceutical companies responsible for supplying new vaccines to the public. Others receive research grant money, funding for their academic departments, or payments for the oversight of vaccine safety trials." "In total, 56 individual patents were found to be owned or shared by one or more members of the ACIP committee or other committees within the CDC." (26) According to the website Justia Patents, the CDC owns at least 200 patents. (27) How many of those have financial ties with vaccines is unsure. Adding to this, "as of 2000, the CDC purchased over half the childhood vaccine administered in the United States through two federally overseen, state-administered programs." (28) The big point here is that the CDC does have some kind of financial gain regarding the increase in the number of vaccines being forced upon our children. That much is perfectly clear.

To illustrate how far the conflicts can go, we can look at the records of a hearing before the Committee on Government Reform House of Representatives. The title of this meeting was FACA: Conflicts of Interest and Vaccine Development--Preserving the Integrity of the Process and was led by Dan Burton of Indiana. In this meeting Mr. Burton brought up six points: "1) that members, including the chair of the FDA and CDC advisory committees who make these decisions own stock in drug companies that make the vaccines. 2) that individuals on both advisory committees own patents for vaccines under consideration, or are affected by the decisions of the committees. 3) that three out of the five of the members of the FDA's advisory committee who voted for the rotavirus vaccine had conflicts of interest that were waived. 4) that 7 individuals of the 15 member FDA advisory committee were not present at the meeting. Two others were excluded from the vote, and the remaining five were joined by five temporary voting members who all voted to license the product. 5) that the CDC grants conflict of interest waivers to every member of their advisory committee a year at a time, and allows full participation in the discussions leading up to a vote by every member, whether they have a financial stake in the decision or not. So they're discussing it, influencing other members possibly, whether they have a financial stake or not. And, 6) that the CDC's advisory committee has no public members, no parents have a vote in whether or not a vaccine belongs on the childhood immunization schedule. The FDA's committee only has one public member." (29)

So even though in 2000 we had congressmen discussing serious conflicts of interest with the CDC nothing seems to change. In 2009 we saw an article titled "Advisers on Vaccines Often Have Conflicts, Report Says" from the *New York Times* reporting more of the same thing. "The report found that 64 percent of the advisers had potential conflicts of interest that were never identified or were left unresolved by the centers. Thirteen percent failed to have an appropriate conflict form on file at the agency at all, which should have barred their participation in the meetings entirely, Mr. Levinson found. And 3 percent voted on matters that ethics officers had already barred them from considering. Most of the advisers identified by Mr. Levinson had either a job or a grant from a company or other entity whose interests were affected by the committees' discussions, and a considerable number also owned stock in such companies, the report said." (30)

In 2016, "a group calling itself CDC Scientists Preserving Integrity, Diligence and Ethics in Research, or (CDC SPIDER), put a list of complaints in writing in a letter to CDC Chief of Staff and provided a copy of the letter to the public watchdog organization U.S. Right to Know (USRTK)." The group stated that, "It appears that our mission is being influenced and shaped by outside parties and rogue interests… and Congressional intent for our agency is being circumvented by some of our leaders. What concerns us most, is that it is becoming the norm and not the rare exception. These questionable and unethical practices threaten to undermine our credibility and reputation as a trusted leader in public health." These whistle-blowing scientists stated that, in regards to a particular large study, "Definitions were changed and data 'cooked' to make the results look better than they were," the complaint states. "An 'internal review' that involved staff across CDC occurred and its findings were essentially suppressed so the media and/or Congressional staff would not become aware of the problems." (31)

If the "SPIDER" group were the only ones talking about this corruption it would be bad enough, however it gets worse. In 2014 another whistle blower had already confessed to major wrongdoing at the CDC. "Dr. William Thompson co-authored four key CDC studies widely touted to exonerate the MMR and vaccines containing the mercury-based preservative, thimerosal, from causing autism. Thompson is a 19 year veteran at the CDC and formerly a senior vaccine safety scientist at their Immunology Safety Office. In August 2014, under Federal whistleblower protection, Dr. Thompson revealed that despite the CDC's claims to the contrary, the vaccine safety studies in question demonstrated a causal link between vaccines and autism symptoms." (32)

Conflicts with the World Health Organization (WHO)

The WHO was established under the charter of the United Nations in 1948. It was originally created to be supported by its member countries (the United States traditionally being one of the largest contributors), however the last few decades have seen a major shift towards private investors. This, not surprisingly, has created very questionable circumstances. Increasing since the 90's, Bill Gates has become the second largest donor to the WHO giving him "an outsized influence" over them. (33) "Kelley Lee, a professor of public health at Simon Fraser University who authored a book about WHO, Lee said the sheer size of the funds from the Gates Foundation compromises WHO's independence. These voluntary contributions are typically earmarked for specific projects or diseases, meaning WHO cannot freely decide how to use them. WHO therefore can't set the global health agenda and has had to do the bidding of rich donors, not only rich nations in Europe and North America, but also rich philanthropies such as the Gates Foundation. 'He who pays the piper plays the tune' as the old saying goes, she said." (33) Another large donor to the WHO are pharmaceutical companies who provide millions of dollars annually. (34) Others are also suggesting that there is even influence from the Ultra Processed Food Industry (UPFI) in WHO decision making in regards to healthy recommendations. (35) Money always increases the chances of corruption and influence over others and the money coming from these sources is incredibly concerning.

One fairly recent criticism of the WHO was their handling of the 2009 H1N1 (bird flu) pandemic. "Among the criticisms was the accusation that the WHO was supporting the pharmaceutical industry by declaring a false pandemic and promoting drugs that increased pharma profits." (36, 37) An article in the *British Medical Journal* stated that "a Europe wide investigation will begin [this week] into the World Health Organization's decision to label the outbreak of swine flu a "pandemic," amid allegations that it did so under pressure from drug companies looking to boost demand for their vaccines." (38) Fiona Godlee, *BMJ* editor-in-chief, was quoted as saying, "Key guidance from WHO—on the need to stockpile antivirals, on the effectiveness of flu vaccines,and on pandemic flu in general—was authored by experts being paid by industry." Harvey Fineberg, President of the Institute of Medicine of the US National Academy of Sciences, also made his doubts clear regarding the WHO's handling of the H1N1 pandemic, "These reports raise questions about potential, inappropriate influences on WHO decision making in the assessment and response to the 2009 H1N1 pandemic and, more generally, question practices employed by WHO to guard against conflict of interest among its expert advisers," he said. (39)

These issues and doubts lead us perfectly into the WHO's handling of the Covid pandemic. Just prior to the pandemic, the WHO had labeled people who refuse to vaccinate as one of their top ten global threats in 2019. Is it simply a coincidence that Covid came along as a perfect vehicle for them to push their vaccine agenda? At the very beginning of the SARs-CoV-2 emergence, even before most countries had decided upon the seriousness of the virus, four organizations came together to "identify potential vaccine makers and to target investments in the development of tests, treatments and shots." One of these four was the Bill & Melinda Gates Foundation, the other three were Gavi, Wellcome Trust and CEPI. Remember, Gates (who either helped found/create or had worked very closely with these other three organizations) is the second largest donor to the WHO. An investigation by POLITICO, stated that this group "used their clout with the World Health Organization to help create an ambitious worldwide distribution plan for the dissemination of those Covid tools to needy nations." POLITICO quoted Lawrence Gostin, a Georgetown University professor who specializes in public-health law as saying, "I think we should be deeply concerned. Putting it in a very crass way, money buys influence. And this is the worst kind of influence."

It was the WHO that was crucial to this groups' rise to power. "All had longstanding ties to the global health body (WHO). The boards of both CEPI and Gavi have a specially designated WHO representative. There is also a revolving door between employment in the groups and work for the WHO: Former WHO employees now work at the Gates Foundation and CEPI; some, such as Chris Wolff, the deputy director of country partnerships at the Gates Foundation, occupy important positions." (40) This very intimate relationship between Gates and the WHO has far too many concerning properties to it. Besides the WHO getting a significant part of its financial contributions from both Gates and from pharmaceutical companies, Gates is in bed with pharma and with the process of manufacturing vaccines in general. Gates has been in the process of making mRNA vaccines since before the Covid pandemic began (41) and was the immediate and largest cheerleader for mRNA vaccines for Covid, even though prior to Covid mRNA vaccines had only produced failed results. (42) Despite this long history of nothing but failed results, Gates came out strong and vocal with his support for the new Covid vaccines, stating in an NBC interview, "everyone who takes the vaccine is not just protecting themselves, but reducing their transmission to other people and allowing society to get back to normal." Two years later he does an about face and states that, "the current vaccines are not infection-blocking. They're not broad, so when new variants come up you lose protection, and they have very short duration, particularly in the people who matter, which are old people." (43) To make these announcements of his even more significant, consider that Gates had purchased large amounts of stock in BioNTech (Pfizer) in 2019, makes his statements telling everyone how wonderful and effective the vaccines are, then in 2021, right before Pfizer's stocks drop dramatically in light of the vaccines poor performance, Gates sells his stock making more than 15 times his original investment. All told, Gates made well over 300 million dollars. (44) And this is someone who has major influence over the WHO.

The last two points I want to mention also have to do with actions taken by the WHO during Covid. The first is the WHO's involvement with censorship. The WHO was in direct communication with Facebook, Instagram, YouTube and Google prior to 2020 to control the information being allowed and being disseminated onto these platforms. (45, 46) Censorship was undoubtedly one of the worst things to reveal its ugly head during the Covid Pandemic and the WHO was right there in the mix. To go along with this idea of suppressing information we should also look at the WHO's investigation of the originof Covid. The WHO sent a hand picked team to investigate the origin of SARs-CoV-2 in 2021. They ultimately decided that a lab leak was an "extremely unlikely pathway." A third of this team had conflicts of interest due to research links or statements, including "Dr. Peter Daszak, president of the EcoHealth Alliance of New York, whose organization funded coronavirus research at the Wuhan Institute of Virology." Another member of the team, Peter Ben Embarek, said during the press conference that the group didn't do "a full investigation or audit" of any particular lab. Overall, he added, the possibility of a lab leak "did not receive the same depth of attention and work" as other hypotheses about the virus' origin." (47, 48) Of course, as we now know the real scoop is that the virus coming from a lab is an extremely LIKELY pathway as the available evidence is now telling us. (49, 50)

Have you seen enough? There is actually a whole lot more on this subject that could be discussed. Should I go on or have I made my case? Can you find corruption in all sorts of places, probably. The problem is we are talking about the system that is responsible for drugs that are being forced upon us and our children. This is the system that is supposed to be protecting our health, not profiting from it. If we can not trust the players within this system, then how on earth are we supposed to trust that the product they are mandating us to have injected into our children is safe and effective. We are dealing with so many layers of corruption that it is near impossible to find any trust in this system at all. And they wonder why more and more people are questioning what they are telling us.

Point Number Six
Unvaccinated are not the cause of outbreaks

"When you blame others, you give up your power to change."
~ Dr. Robert Anthony, Author

Let me clarify something, can an unvaccinated person be the cause of an outbreak of "something?" Of course they can. The point with this "point" is... so can vaccinated individuals. The source of an outbreak of whatever disease we are discussing can come from either vaccinated or unvaccinated. The major issue goes back to information discussed in Point Three: Media Bias and Censorship. If there is an outbreak it is guaranteed to be reported in the media as being caused by an unvaccinated child. Even when the media does mention that most or all of the people in an outbreak were vaccinated, they still somehow bring the conversation back around to the unvaccinated and how they are the ones responsible and need to get vaccinated to help protect others. They continue to reinforce the false narrative. It is further evidence of the bias and censorship regarding vaccine information. If it was honest reporting, honest information, then we would hear the media giving accurate and balanced information as opposed to a completely one sided narrative. The media would accurately report how many were vaccinated in a given outbreak instead of simply saying there is an outbreak and it was caused by the unvaccinated. Integrating these immunological findings into outbreak narratives would provide a more balanced understanding of vaccine and disease dynamics. For example, pathogenic priming, where the immune system's preconditioning by vaccines may inadvertently worsen responses to pathogens, is rarely presented in the media, but is critical for assessing overall public health strategies that include consideration of vaccine risks and benefits.

The simple fact that there is ample evidence of outbreaks beginning in fully vaccinated populations that never gets discussed by the media clearly illustrates their deliberate bias in this matter. Emerging research into immunological phenomena such as molecular mimicry, offers further insight into these outbreaks. Studies, including Vojdani et al.'s validation of pathogenic priming, have shown that vaccine-induced immune responses can, in rare cases, lead to cross-reactivity with host tissues. This mechanism may exacerbate disease severity or contribute to atypical immune responses, complicating assumptions about immunity and outbreak dynamics. (1) Consider the following quote "Some states are engaging in such wide exemptions that they're creating the opportunity for outbreaks on a scale that is going to have national implications," Scott Gottlieb, the head of the FDA from 2017-2019. (2) This comment was made in response to outbreaks of measles in 2019. The article by CNBC never once mentions the fact that measles outbreaks can, have and do occur in fully vaccinated populations all the time. They simply go on to talk about how it is so terrible that people go unvaccinated and how states are proposing legislation to take away a person's right to refuse vaccines. Don't even bother to mention that these same vaccines that are going to then be forced on individuals can still produce the outbreaks that they are complaining about. Measles is the perfect virus to illustrate this point regarding vaccinated outbreaks and the ridiculous one-sided reporting that occurs around it. Check out the conclusion that this article from the prestigious *New England Journal of Medicine* in 1985 titled "Measles Outbreak in a Fully Immunized Secondary-School Population" came to, "We conclude that outbreaks of measles can occur in secondary schools, even when more than 99 percent of the students have been vaccinated and more than 95 percent are immune." (3)

This next point of information is taken directly from the CDC: "In 1978, the CDC set a goal to eliminate measles from the United States by 1982. Although this goal was not met, widespread use of the measles vaccine drastically reduced the disease rates. By 1981, the number of reported measles cases was 80% less compared with the previous year. However, a 1989 measles outbreaks among vaccinated school-aged children prompted the Advisory Committee on

Practices (ACIP), the American Academy of Pediatrics (AAP), and the American Academy of Family Physicians (AAFP) to recommend a second dose of MMR vaccine for all children." (4)

In an article in the *Canadian Journal of Public Health* titled, "Major measles epidemic in the region of Quebec despite a 99% vaccine coverage," it was stated that "The vaccination coverage among cases was at least 84.5%. Vaccination coverage for the total population was 99.0%." (5) They went on to state that "Incomplete vaccination coverage is not a valid explanation for the Quebec City measles outbreak." This incidence also occurred in 1989 around the same time as the outbreak in the U.S. So the second dose that was added to the schedule in 1989-90 was supposed to fix this problem, right? This next article is also regarding Quebec but the year is 2011. Coming from *The Journal of Infectious Diseases* and titled, "Largest Measles Epidemic in North America in a Decade..." Here they state, "The largest measles epidemic in North America in the last decade, occurred in 2011 in Quebec, Canada, where rates of 1- and 2-dose vaccine coverage among children 3 years of age were 95%–97% and 90%" So according to this article, upwards of 97% had one shot and 90% had two, yet there was still an outbreak. They went on to conclude that, "Unvaccinated individuals remain the immunization priority, but a better understanding of susceptibility in 2-dose recipients is needed to define effective interventions if elimination is to be achieved." (6) Interesting how, even with the outbreak clearly showing the ineffectiveness of the vaccine to prevent the outbreak, they still felt the need to focus on the very small percent of those that were unvaccinated.

In an article from *The Journal of Clinical Infectious Disease* titled, Outbreak of measles among persons with prior evidence of immunity, New York City, 2011 "the first report of measles transmission from a twice-vaccinated individual with documented secondary vaccine failure." (7) Here is another article straight from the CDC titled, "Measles Outbreak Associated with Vaccine Failure in Adults." Here they stated, "Approximately two thirds of cases occurred among adults, most of whom had received ≥1 dose of MCV, with many receiving 2 doses." (8) This occurred in 2014. In an article in the *Journal of Clinical*

Microbiology they showed that "Of the 194 measles virus sequences obtained in the United States in 2015, 73 were identified as vaccine sequences." (9) That is, 38% of all measles cases in 2015 were vaccinated. If you were to take out the number of children that were too young to have been vaccinated in the first place (which would increase the vaccinated percentage) you begin to see how this is not an unvaccinated issue.

How about other vaccine related diseases:

This article came from the *LA Times* and is a perfect example of the media focusing a vaccinated outbreak back onto those who choose not to vaccinate. The article titled "Harvard-Westlake students were vaccinated. Dozens caught whooping cough anyway" stated that "all 90 people who have recently come down with pertussis — the official name for whooping cough — in Los Angeles County this year had been immunized against it, according to county officials." However the chief medical officer at USC Verdugo Hills Hospital said that even though the vaccine's immunity wanes, increasing coverage rates in the community would help prevent pertussis outbreaks. Once there's a chink in the armor and that unvaccinated population grows, then the actual protection of the vaccination significantly drops, even for those who are vaccinated." (10) Question, if the vaccine is supposed to protect a person from contracting pertussis and obviously did not do its job...how does my vaccine status affect that? The only chink in the armor that I can see here is their own vaccine. This next paper comes from the prestigious *New England Journal of Medicine* and is titled "The 1993 Epidemic of Pertussis in Cincinnati -- Resurgence of Disease in a Highly Immunized Population of Children." "Immunization records revealed that 74 percent (75 of 101) of the children with pertussis who were 19 months to 12 years old had received four or five doses of the combined diphtheria-pertussis-tetanus (DPT) vaccine, and that 82 percent (103 of 126) of those 7 to 71 months old had received at least three doses of DPT vaccine." (11) Please pay attention to the fact that these children had between 3 and five doses of DPT vaccine and were still contracting whooping cough.

To add even more chinks to the pertussis vaccines "armor" comes this great article from *CIDRAP* (The Center for Infectious Disease Research and Policy) titled "Whooping cough cases tied to waning vaccine protection." Check out what they found here, "The researchers identified 738 pertussis cases, with 99 cases in unvaccinated children, 36 in undervaccinated children, 515 in fully vaccinated children (five DTaP doses), and 88 in children who had received six doses of DTaP." (12) Not only were 515 fully vaccinated but 88 had received six doses and still caught whooping cough! I think their armor has more than just a few chinks in it (just say'n).

How about mumps?

This is from a journal called *European Surveillance* and the article is titled, "Waning immunity against mumps in vaccinated young adults, France 2013," "15 clusters of mumps were notified in France; 72% (82/114) of the cases had been vaccinated twice with measles-mumps-rubella vaccine." (13) From the journal *Vaccine*, "Mumps resurgences in the United States: A historical perspective on unexpected elements," "In 2006 the United States experienced the largest nationwide mumps epidemic in 20 years, primarily affecting college dormitory residents (63% of case-patients had received two doses)." (14) Here's one more for mumps from the *Journal of Clinical Infectious Disease,* this article is titled "Mumps vaccine performance among university students during a mumps outbreak," "High 2-dose MMR coverage protected many students from developing mumps but was not sufficient to prevent the mumps outbreak. Vaccine-induced protection may wane." (15) Finally let's round out the MMR vaccine with this one regarding rubella from the journal *California Medicine* titled "Transmission of rubella vaccine virus from vaccinees to contacts," "The report presents evidence of the transmission of hpv-77 derived rubella vaccine virus from vaccinees to two susceptible contacts.(16)"

But wait...we're not finished.

Here are a couple of articles regarding the influenza vaccine. This first one from the *Journal of Clinical Infectious Disease* titled, "Influenza Vaccine Effectiveness in the Community and the Household," "Substantially lower effectiveness was noted among subjects who were vaccinated in both the current and prior season. There was no evidence that vaccination prevented household transmission once influenza was introduced; adults were at particular risk despite vaccination." (17) Our last article is another straight from the CDC titled "Influenza Outbreak in a Vaccinated Population — USS Ardent, February 2014," "despite vaccination measures, influenza outbreaks can still occur in highly vaccinated military populations." (18)

How about the much lauded Polio vaccine? Look at this paper from the *Lancet* in 1991 titled "Outbreak of paralytic poliomyelitis in Oman: evidence for widespread transmission among fully vaccinated children," "From January, 1988, to March, 1989, a widespread outbreak (118 cases) of poliomyelitis type 1 occurred in Oman." "...a substantial proportion of fully vaccinated children had been involved in the chain of transmission."(19)

Vaccine "failure" is not a fringe idea but is a widely known situation already discussed by researchers. This article written in the journal *Vaccine* titled "A framework for research on vaccine effectiveness," (20) does an excellent job discussing some of the current theories regarding vaccine failure. The authors make the straight forward assessment that "vaccines are typically very effective but rarely provide permanent and complete protection from infection." There were five reasons they cited for "vaccine failure." Those being:

1. Primary vaccine failure is the occurrence of infection or disease in a fully vaccinated individual who failed to make an immune response to the vaccine

2. Secondary vaccine failure is the occurrence of infection or disease in a fully vaccinated individual who made a normal immune response to the vaccine (which may or may not have been measured) but whose immunity has subsequently waned.

3. "Exposure threshold" vaccines in which VE (vaccine effectiveness) depends on the dose of exposure and is lower following high dose exposure than low dose exposure

4. "Leaky vaccines" in which each exposure carries an equal risk of infection for everyone, with no change in severity; may look like waning after multiple exposures

5. Multimodal in which multiple modes of action (and/or vaccine failure) co-exist

The one common denominator among all of the discussions regarding vaccine failure is that those involved never seem to move beyond their story of vaccines for all. They still stick to the party line that vaccines are always good and everyone should have to take them. There are many questions that this should be bringing up...

1. If I can, not only catch the disease I am being vaccinated for through the vaccine itself, but can also spread the disease for which the vaccine is supposed to prevent, then why should I be forced to take the vaccine?

2. If I can, not only catch the disease I am being vaccinated for through the vaccine itself, but can also spread the disease for which the vaccine is supposed to prevent, then why are the media and the "experts" constantly pointing their respective fingers at the unvaccinated?

3. If I can, not only catch the disease I am being vaccinated for through the vaccine itself, but can also spread the disease for which the vaccine is supposed to prevent, then why should I choose to take a vaccine for what are mostly non-life threatening diseases?

4. If I can, not only catch the disease I am being vaccinated for through the vaccine itself, but can also spread the disease for which the vaccine is supposed to prevent, then why should I

risk unknown (and known) problems from vaccines for diseases that are mostly non-life threatening? (see Point 7)

5. If I can, not only catch the disease I am being vaccinated for through the vaccine itself, but can also spread the disease for which the vaccine is supposed to prevent, then why doesn't the media discuss this or even allow for open discussion regarding vaccines at all?

I am sure we could come up with more questions to ask. Bottom line, outbreaks of disease are not exclusively linked to the unvaccinated. In many cases the outbreaks are stemming from populations of fully vaccinated individuals. This is not an opinion, but a proven fact.

Point Number Seven
Vaccines are Not "perfectly safe"

According to Merriam-Webster online dictionary the word safe can be defined in two of the following ways:

1. "not able or likely to be hurt or harmed in any way : not in danger"
2. "not involving or likely to involve danger, harm, or loss" (1)

If you do even a cursory search into the subject of vaccines, one statement that you will see repeated over and over again in various forms is that vaccines are safe and effective. News agencies tend to use this statement in their reports as some kind of known fact that should reassure their readers or listeners. "Don't worry about what any of those 'anti-vaxxers' say because vaccines are proven to be 'safe and effective." For example:

- According to The American Academy of Family Physicians Foundation: "Vaccines Are Safe, Effective and Save Lives."(2)
- UNICEF states that, "Vaccines are very safe." (3)
- The National Academies of Science and Engineering Medicine goes one-step further by adding the word 'extremely' to their claim "Vaccines are extremely safe."(4)
- The CDC wants you to know that when it comes to vaccines, "the final product is safe and effective." (5)
- And according to the World Health Organization: "Vaccination is safe and side effects from a vaccine are usually minor and temporary, such as a sore arm or mild fever. More serious side effects are possible, but extremely rare." (6)

Despite repeated assurances from public health authorities that vaccines are 'safe and effective,' the US Supreme Court in a 2011 acknowledged Congress's classification of vaccines as "unavoidably unsafe." (7) (This phrase was taken from the National Vaccine Injury

Act of 1986 and was essentially used as a way to help insure their protection against liability.) And then there is this statement taken from The Committee on Government Reform in 2000, "Every year, a number of children are seriously injured by adverse reactions to vaccines. When such a tragedy befalls a family, they are faced with devastating emotional and financial consequences. As the devastation of adverse reactions can lead to paralysis, permanent disability and death, families without adequate insurance can face enormous expenses, including residential care, therapy, medical equipment, and drugs."(8) So on the one hand you have all manner of news agencies, and scientific and government agencies uniformly stating that vaccines are safe and then on the other hand you have Congress stating quite plainly that all vaccines are "unavoidably unsafe." So which is it?

What follows are portions of a timeline that was taken from a website called History of Vaccines (an award-winning informational, educational website created by The College of Physicians of Philadelphia). (9) Other sources have also been inserted into this timeline to attempt to make it even more accurate:

- 1901 Contaminated smallpox vaccine leads to tetanus outbreak; 13 children died.
- 1901 children die from contaminated diphtheria antitoxin
- 1916 In Columbia, South Carolina, a tainted batch of typhoid vaccine stored at room temperature caused 68 severe reactions, 26 abscesses, and 4 deaths. (10)
- 1919 Dallas Disaster, five children die from contaminated diphtheria vaccine
- 1925 Children die from failed whooping cough vaccine (11)
- 1928 Queensland Disaster, 12 of 21 children die from diphtheria vaccine (10)
- 1929 Lubeck Disaster, 72 babies die from TB vaccine
- 1935 Early polio vaccine trials prove a disaster. Kills or paralyzes many test subjects.
- 1942 Several deaths and thousands of cases of liver damage following hepatitis vaccination of Army troops.
- 1947 The first published reports appear of irreversible brain damage after whole-cell pertussis vaccine (11)

- 1952 The Cutter Incident, polio vaccine causes 40,000 cases of polio leaving 200 children paralyzed and 10 dead
- 1959 The Parke-Davis Quadrigen vaccine (DPT combined with the Salk polio vaccine) is licensed. The vaccine is alleged to be particularly reactive because of the effect of the preservative on the pertussis component. Several lawsuits ensue. The vaccine was withdrawn from the market in 1968 (11)
- 1960 Polio vaccines found to be contaminated with SV40 from monkey cells (SV40 is now a known link to many cancers still occuring today) (13)(14)(15)
- 1969-1976 Reports of possible serious adverse events following rubella vaccination began to be published. Two types of events are reported: neuropathies and acute and chronic arthralgia and arthritis. (11)
- 1969 An experimental formalin-inactivated vaccine led to more severe RSV disease (with two deaths) (16)
- 1974 In Great Britain, questions about the safety of whole-cell pertussis vaccines are widely publicized in the popular press after newspaper accounts of a study (Kulenkampff et al., 1974) suggesting adverse reactions. (11)
- 1975 Japan temporarily stops using the pertussis vaccine after publicity about deaths following vaccination.(11)
- 1976 After mass vaccination with the Swine flu vaccine, more than 500 cases of GuillainBarre syndrome occurred among the vaccinated persons, with 25 deaths.(17) (18)
- 1978 Two lawsuits are filed in U.S. courts alleging that children were harmed by pertussis vaccine (11)
- 1979-1980's Systematic investigations are undertaken for the possible association between rubella vaccines and chronic arthritis or arthropathies, leading to an increased level of concern on the part of some investigators (11)
- 1981 Cody et al. finds higher reactions in DTP versus DT vaccine. Following DTP immunization nine children in the study developed convulsions and nine developed hypotonic hyporesponsive episodes.
- 1981 NCES study, "The evidence is consistent with a causal relation between DPT and acute encephalopathy"(11)(12)

- 1985 A total of 219 lawsuits were filed in U.S. courts alleging harm to a child from the pertussis vaccine. The average amount of compensation sought (when specified) is $26 million. (11)
- 1986 The National Childhood Vaccine Injury Act (VICP), is passed by the U.S. Congress. This act gives vaccine manufacturers immunity from prosecution from any lawsuits pertaining to vaccine injury. (11)
- 1991 CDC is considering issuing a request for proposals for a study of chronic arthritis following rubella vaccination (11)
- 1991 Gulf War Syndrome possibly linked to anthrax vaccine(18)
- 1998 Myofasciitis linked to aluminum in vaccines (18)
- 1999 Rotavirus vaccine removed from use over potentially fatal bowel problems
- 2010-12 After vaccination with Pandemrix (a vaccine for H1N1) 761 case reports of narcolepsy (confirmed and unconfirmed) following vaccination.(18)(19)
- 2018 attorneys negotiated a $101 million settlement for an infant who suffered a severe reaction (a severe brain injury, encephalopathy, cortical vision impairment, truncal hypotonia (low muscle tone), and kidney failure.) to the MMR vaccine.(20)
- 2024 Covid vaccines are under the microscope for myocarditis and other problems. Only time will tell what else comes from these vaccines.

One incident that did not make it into my timeline comes from a research article that took about 30 years to see the light of day. Titled "The Introduction of Diphtheria-Tetanus-Pertussis and Oral Polio Vaccine Among Young Infants in an Urban African Community: A Natural Experiment" and published in *eBioMedicine* (part of the *Lancet*), what the researchers reported was nothing short of startling, " All currently available evidence suggests that DTP vaccine may kill more children from other causes than it saves from diphtheria, tetanus or pertussis. Though a vaccine protects children against the target disease it may simultaneously increase susceptibility to unrelated infections." (21) Another study involving the DTP vaccine had a similar finding, "Receipt of DTP (almost always with oral polio vaccine) was associated with a possible increase in all cause mortality on average (relative risk 1.38, 0.92 to 2.08) from 10 studies at high risk of bias; this effect seemed stronger in girls than in boys."(22) We are definitely looking at "unavoidably unsafe" at this point in our discussion.

From the website vaccinelaw.com, attorney Leah Durant writes: "Each year, hundreds of individuals file claims with the National Vaccine Injury Compensation Program (VICP), and these claimants represent only a small fraction of the vaccine recipients who experience pain and other symptoms as a result of their vaccinations." According to this attorney, who specializes in vaccine injuries, the two most common injuries are shoulder injury related to vaccine administration (SIRVA) and Guillain-Barre Syndrome (GBS). (23) Another vaccine injury law group goes even further. They also list SIRVA and GBS but include allergic reactions, autoimmune disorders, blood conditions, bowel problems, nerve damage and pain and even brain injuries. (24) If this list of potential injuries alarms you then you should take a look at the complete Vaccine Injury Table created by the Health Resources & Services Administration (HRSA). (25) The most current Table is from 2017 and contains far more injuries than either of these two lawyers discuss on their websites.

Far more alarming is the information uncovered by the Institutes of Medicine (IOM) reports. "In 1991, the Institutes of Medicine (IOM) examined 22 commonly reported serious injuries following the DTP vaccine. The IOM concluded the scientific literature supported a causal relationship between the DTP vaccine and 6 of these injuries: acute encephalopathy, chronic arthritis, acute arthritis, shock and unusual shock-like state, anaphylaxis, and protracted inconsolable crying. The IOM, however, found the scientific literature was insufficient to conclude whether or not the DTP vaccine can cause 12 other serious injuries. The IOM lamented that it "encountered many gaps and limitations in knowledge bearing directly and indirectly on the safety of vaccines" and on the poor design of the few existing studies. It therefore cautioned that: "If research capacity and accomplishment in this field are not improved, future reviews of vaccine safety will be similarly handicapped." In 1994, the IOM issued another report which examined the scientific literature for evidence that could either prove or disprove a causal link between 54 commonly reported serious injuries and vaccination for diphtheria, tetanus, measles, mumps, polio, hepatitis B, and Hib. The IOM located sufficient science to support a causal connection between these vaccines and 12 injuries, including death, anaphylaxis, thrombocytopenia, and Guillain-Barre syndrome. The IOM, however, found the scientific literature was insufficient to conclude whether or not these vaccines caused 38 other commonly reported serious injuries.

As in 1991, this IOM Report again stated, "The lack of adequate data regarding many of the adverse events under study was of major concern to the committee. Presentations at public meetings indicated that many parents and physicians share this concern." In 2011, more than fifteen years after the IOM Reports in 1991 and 1994, HHS paid the IOM to conduct another assessment regarding vaccine safety. This third IOM Report reviewed the available science with regard to the 158 most common vaccine injuries claimed to have occurred from vaccination for varicella, hepatitis B, tetanus, measles, mumps, and rubella. The IOM located science which "convincingly supports a causal relationship" with 14 of these injuries, including pneumonia, meningitis, hepatitis, MIBE, febrile seizures, and anaphylaxis. The review found sufficient evidence to support "acceptance of a causal relationship" with four additional serious injuries. The IOM, however, found the scientific literature was insufficient to conclude whether or not those vaccines caused 135 other serious injuries commonly reported after their administration.

Thus, out of the 158 most common serious injuries reported to have been caused by the vaccines under review, the evidence supported a causal relationship for 18 of them, rejected a causal relationship for five of them, but for the remaining 135 vaccine-injury pairs, over 86 percent of those reviewed, the IOM found that the science simply had not been performed." (26) What's truly alarming here is not what was confirmed to be caused by the vaccines, but the incredible number of possible injuries/conditions that do not have enough evidence to confirm or deny the connections. And the fact that over the 15 years between the IOM's reviews, nothing was ever done to discover if there even is a connection to those vaccine injuries. As they stated in their report "the science had simply not been performed."

Not only is the science "not being performed," but also when studies are performed they are not always done in a manner that would give valid results that would inform us as to the vaccines safety. For example, many vaccines are not tested utilizing what the science community states as the "gold standard." Here is what the National Institutes of Health (NIH) has to say regarding testing, "In undertaking a clinical trial, researchers don't want to leave anything to chance. They want to be as certain as possible that the results of the testing show whether or not a treatment is safe and effective. The "gold standard" for testing interventions in people is the randomized, placebo-controlled clinical trial. That means volunteers are randomly assigned—that is, selected by chance—to either a test group receiving the experimental intervention or a control group receiving a placebo or standard care. A placebo is an inactive substance that looks like the drug or treatment being tested." (27) While many vaccines have used a true placebo (saline only) in their trials, there are still more that state they are using a placebo, when in fact they are utilizing something that is not at all an "inactive substance." (28)(29)(30)(31)(32)(33) Some of these studies have used another vaccine as the placebo or they use a shot containing all of the ingredients of the test vaccine excluding the antigen. There is no way possible to assess the safety of a vaccine if what you are comparing it to has the same possible side effects. If you do a study in this manner you can easily say at the end of the study that the vaccine being tested was no more harmful than the placebo. It is easy to say when the "placebo" is also something that is also potentially harmful.

Those who are charged with defending vaccines will say that it is unethical to perform a test on a vaccine with a true placebo. They will try to tell you that because vaccines are proven to be safe and effective, and that they save lives; denying the vaccine to all of the participants in a trial is not ethical and potentially places participants at risk if they are not getting the vaccine.(34) If a drug company took this approach with all of their drug studies (our drug saves lives therefore denying it to any participant in the study is unethical) then every drug produced would have no safety testing prior to release. All medications would have nothing to compare themselves to. Vaccines are classified as biologics, not drugs, but this should not then entitle them to be treated any differently in their research process. It is just as important, if not more so, that vaccines be held to the same standard as any other drug being researched. I would argue that it is even more important to be accurate and ethical as vaccines are the only drugs that are being mandated. Comparison with an actual placebo is paramount if we are to have any hope of being able to detect harmful effects.

Beyond whether or not the research is done in an honest and ethical manner, the end result is a pharmaceutical product. The notion that vaccines are somehow the one and only pharmaceutical product that we never need to worry about is farcical. Researchers are very familiar with the seriousness of this issue, "it is well recognised that numerous side effects are not observed during clinical trials but are only identified after the drug has reached the market. For this reason, drug side effects remain a leading cause of morbidity and mortality in healthcare, with an annual loss of billions of dollars." (35) Add into this equation the fact that pharmaceutical companies have no liability with vaccines and the farce becomes downright scary.

The only real method we have for assessing the safety of vaccines is the Vaccine Adverse Reporting System (VAERS). "Established in 1990, the Vaccine Adverse Event Reporting System (VAERS) is a national early warning system to detect possible safety problems in U.S.-licensed vaccines. VAERS is co-managed by the Centers for Disease Control and Prevention (CDC) and the U.S. Food and Drug Administration (FDA). VAERS accepts and analyzes reports of adverse events (possible side effects) after a person has received a vaccination. Anyone can report an adverse event to VAERS. Healthcare professionals are required to report certain adverse events and vaccine manufacturers are required to report all adverse events that come to their attention." "VAERS is a passive reporting system, meaning it relies on individuals to send in reports of their experiences to CDC and FDA. VAERS is not designed to determine if a vaccine caused a health problem, but is especially useful for detecting unusual or unexpected patterns of adverse event reporting that might indicate a possible safety problem with a vaccine. This way, VAERS can provide CDC and FDA with valuable information that additional work and evaluation is necessary to further assess a possible safety concern." (36)

Once again from The Committee on Government Reform, "While the Vaccine Adverse Events Reporting System [VAERS] may be lauded as the "front line" of vaccine safety, the lack of enforcement provisions and effective monitoring of reporting practices preclude accurate assessments of the extent to which adverse events are actually reported. Former FDA Commissioner David A. Kessler has estimated that VAERS reports currently represent only a fraction of the serious adverse events. The quality of VAERS data has been questioned. Because reports are submitted from a variety of sources, some inexperienced in completing data forms for medical studies, many reports omit important data and contain obvious errors. Assessment is further complicated by the administration of multiple vaccines at the same time, following currently recommended vaccine schedules, because there may be no conclusive way to determine which vaccine or combination of vaccines caused the specific adverse event. As a database for epidemiological studies, VAERS has serious weaknesses. One major problem is that since unvaccinated people experiencing adverse events are not reported to VAERS, there is no control group to study. Given that over 10,000 reports are filed annually, it is difficult to assure the accuracy and completeness of the database." (8) This notion of underreporting of vaccine adverse events was brought home in a study done in 2009 by a research arm of Harvard. Here they confirmed what the FDA commissioner mentioned in the above statement, "Likewise, fewer than 1% of vaccine adverse events are reported." (37)

The National Vaccine Injury Compensation Program, which was created in 1986, is a no-fault alternative to the traditional tort system. It provides compensation to people found to be injured by certain vaccines.(38) Whereas "the VICP compensates people whose injuries may have been caused by certain vaccines. The program is separate from VAERS, and administered by the Health Resources and Service Administration. Reporting an adverse event to VAERS does not create a claim for compensation with the VICP. Claims must be filed separately with the VICP." (39) VAERS may be "separate" from VICP, yet it is VAERS that is supposed to alert the regulatory agencies of potential issues regarding individual vaccines. Once alerted to potential issues, these agencies can go about the task of investigating the issues. If the reported issues are proven to be accurate, these new injuries will then be added to something called the Vaccine Injury Table. The Vaccine Injury Table is what is used in the VICP process for claimants to be able to prove their injury case. If their injury is not on this table their case becomes much harder to win. The problem is, if this reporting system is only capturing 1% of adverse events then these agencies are not getting the full picture of the potential harm from the vaccines. Even if the information regarding the 1% was inaccurate and it was say closer to 10% or even 40%, it would still mean that the record of injuries from vaccines is far higher than is being reported to these agencies or to the public. So even with a reporting system that is this dysfunctional and even with a process that the vast majority of Americans know nothing about (40); since the inception of the VICP, total compensation to victims of vaccine injury (so far) is 4.7 billion dollars. (41) Imagine what that number would possibly be if adverse vaccine events were being recorded accurately? Just look at the difference in reporting if we take into consideration the discrepancies we have mentioned already. If we look at the deaths reported to VAERS from 1997-2013 which were 2,149 (42) and we then assume that this is only 1% of the actual number, then this would put the actual number of deaths that may have occurred at well over 200,000. Imagine the conversation if this was the actual number? The problem is, that with a reporting system that is not collecting the correct data we will never know.

I think I have sufficiently illustrated that there is absolutely a big question regarding vaccine safety, however I want to throw in a few other issues from the scientific literature to add to this question of vaccine safety. The question of a possible link between sudden infant death syndrome (SIDS) and vaccines has been a persistent issue for well over fifty years. Multiple studies have discussed that there is no causal link between SIDS and DTP vaccination yet most of these same studies admit that there is a definitive temporal association. There are also plenty of other studies that still insist on a connection between the two. (43)(44)(45)(46) One such study said this regarding the connection, "Judgment of the disorders as truly related to vaccination is difficult, but suspicious cases do exist. Forensic pathologists must devote more attention to vaccination in sudden infant death cases."(46) We already know that the DTP vaccine can cause "significant neurological illness" (47) so is it really a stretch to connect the DTP shot to something like SIDS? Having found at least one verifiable court case that shows vaccines as a factor in the death of a five month old boy from SIDS I would say there is not much of a stretch necessary. (48)

Another point of interest, if you go back to the timeline and look at 1960, you will see the information on SV40 contamination in polio vaccines and their link to cancers. Sv40 is also now being linked to other conditions as well. In a paper titled Serum antibodies from epileptic patients react, at high prevalence, with simian virus 40 mimotopes the authors made this conclusion, "Our immunological data suggest a strong association between epilepsy and the SV40 infection."(49) A similar finding was made in another paper, "Simian virus and other viruses causing encephalitis may result in super-refractory status epilepticus (SRSE)."(50) Besides the already known link between SV40 and a whole list of cancers there are even findings of a possible link between the SV40 contamination and multiple sclerosis and with kidney disease (51)(52) The most humorous (and by humorous I mean not humorous) thing about SV40 is the following statement from another paper, "It is of no small irony that SV40, once having been found as an unrecognized contaminant of a widely heralded viral vaccine, might itself one day become a candidate for vaccine development."(53) And somehow the vaccine manufacturers wonder why some people suspect them of creating new problems to make money off of?

Lastly, it is widely known among the science community that the prevalence of autoimmune diseases has been increasing steadily for sometime.(54) The possible link between vaccines and this situation is becoming clearer as is shown in the following statement, "The autoimmune/inflammatory syndrome induced by adjuvants (ASIA) is a recently identified condition in which the exposure to an adjuvant leads to an aberrant immune response." (55) In fact many researchers are well aware of the connection, "Vaccines have been suspected of playing a role in inducing autoimmune disease (AID) for a long time." (56) These researchers are already understanding some of the mechanisms that may be involved as shown from this quote, "Among the implicated mechanisms for these reactions is molecular mimicry. Molecular mimicry refers to a significant similarity between certain pathogenic elements contained in the vaccine and specific human proteins. This similarity may lead to immune cross-reactivity, wherein the reaction of the immune system towards the pathogenic antigens may harm the similar human proteins, essentially causing autoimmune disease."(57) These reactions have already been confirmed in the recent COVID-19 vaccinations. (58)(59)

I think we should throw in the following information, that is in regards to adverse reactions from drugs in general, just to get an even better look at the scope of what we are involved with here. This information is taken from the FDA: "The first question healthcare providers should ask themselves is "why is it important to learn about ADRs?" The answer is because ADRs are one of the leading causes of morbidity and mortality in health care. The Institute of Medicine reported in January of 2000 that between 44,000 to 98,000 deaths occur annually from medical errors. Of this total, an estimated 7,000 deaths occur due to ADRs. However, other studies conducted on hospitalized patient populations have placed much higher estimates on the overall incidence of serious ADRs. These studies estimate that 6.7% of hospitalized patients have a serious adverse drug reaction with a fatality rate of 0.32%. If these estimates are correct, then there are more than 2,216,000 serious ADRs in hospitalized patients, causing over 106,000 deaths annually. If true, then ADRs are the 4th leading cause of death—ahead of pulmonary disease, diabetes, AIDS, pneumonia, accidents, and automobile deaths. These statistics do not include the number of ADRs that occur in ambulatory settings. Also, it is estimated that over 350,000 ADRs occur in U.S. nursing homes each year. The exact number of ADRs is not certain and is limited by methodological considerations. However, whatever the true numberis, ADRs represent a significant public health problem that is, for the most part, preventable." (59) Are we really expected to believe that this is true for all medications, yet vaccines are immune to these same problems?

The science community, pharmaceutical companies and our government all know that vaccines are "unavoidably unsafe." They all know that some very serious adverse events can be caused by vaccines, including death. They also are all completely aware that whatever it is they may think they understand about these adverse events, it is likely far more serious than the current data suggests since our methods for tracking these events are not adequate. Yet all of these groups do not perform the necessary steps to uncover the facts, make necessary changes or even share truthful information to the media and to the public. It is perfectly logical as to why they do not do these things... money. Can you fathom what the consequences will be once the public becomes fully aware of the actual harms caused by vaccines? If they have already paid out four billion dollars for the fraction of harms that have been able to squeak through the system created by the regulatory agencies, how much will they have to pay out once the reality of vaccine damage becomes common knowledge? Furthermore, how much revenue will they lose once more Americans understand the game of Russian Roulette they are playing when they decide to give their children these vaccines. And, if we make this information known then how on earth can any of these vaccines be mandated? If any person still wishes to take vaccines after understanding all of the potential consequences then that is their right, however if after understanding this information they decide not to take the vaccines that is also their choice. This is the choice that we are discussing here. It is the choice that so many have been fighting for and it is the purpose of all of the information you will find contained in these pages.

Point Number Eight
Vaccines and Autism

"I think that the public health officials have been too quick to dismiss the hypothesis [that vaccines cause autism] as irrational."
~Bernadine Healy, M.D., the first woman to direct the National Institutes of Health (NIH)

Is there a more contentious topic when it comes to vaccines then the dreaded, "Do vaccines cause autism?" I don't think that there is. This is like the Holy Grail of vaccine topics. It certainly is the topic that the vaccine apologists love to come back to as their point for driving home the "science" of how the "anti-vaxxers" are so wrong about everything involved in denying vaccines. This is another of the many subjects that has a very specific script which it seems every media outlet likes to read from. It typically goes something like this, "There is no connection between vaccines and autism." How about some examples:

- "there is no connection between vaccines and autism." kidshealth.org/en/parents/autism-studies.html
- "There is no correlation between autism and vaccines." autismsciencefoundation.org/autism-and-vaccines/
- "Vaccines do not cause autism." "Vaccine ingredients do not cause autism." (since updated 2025) www.cdc.gov/vaccinesafety/concerns/autism.html
- "The research is clear: Vaccines don't cause autism." www.webmd.com/brain/autism/do-vaccines-cause-autism
- "Evidence Shows Vaccines Unrelated to Autism" www.immunize.org/catg.d/p4028.pdf

"no link between vaccines and autism." healthy.kaiserpermanente.org/health-wellness/health-encyclopedia/he.autism-and-vaccines.ue4907

I could go on for pages with more of the exact same denials. The script is that study after study has proven that there is no correlation between vaccines and autism and that anyone saying differently is just denying the science. An interesting thing with that statement is what they really mean or should be saying, is that there is no correlation between the MMR vaccine and autism. To be even more accurate they would have to state that there is no correlation between thimerosal and autism. Their response to issues over vaccine concerns is very reactionary and it appears to be that their only objective is damage control. You see, instead of actually making a real attempt to see if there is an actual correlation between vaccines and autism, those in charge take the one thing that opponents have made an accusation about (MMR and Thimerosal) and decide to show that they are wrong. Now any time the question comes up, do vaccines cause autism? They say, no they do not and we've proven it, however as stated, that is not what their science actually shows. What we should be asking is why are they far more interested in defending their vaccine program then they are finding real answers.

First, let's look at autism and why it is such a concern. "Autism was once considered a rare disease that affected an estimated 1 in 10,000 individuals in the United States. The Committee [on Government Reform] held its first hearing on the dramatic rise in autism in April of 2000. At the time, Federal agencies were estimating that autism affected 1 in 500 children in the United States. By 2002, the National Institutes of Health had adjusted that rate to 1 in 250 children in the United States. The Autism Society of America estimates that the number of autistic children is growing by 10 to 17 percent each year." "A study on autism in California determined that the number of autistic individuals in that state has nearly tripled. Equally important, the study stated that the increase was real, and could not be explained by changes in diagnostic criteria or better diagnoses."(1) "In 2021, the CDC reported that approximately 1 in 44 children in the U.S. is diagnosed with an autism spectrum disorder (ASD), according to 2018 data." "Boys are four times more likely to be diagnosed with autism than girls."(2) As you can see, the number of children with ASD has been rising exponentially since the 1990's. From an estimated 1 in 10,000 individuals to now more than 1 in 23 in the U.S. all occurring since the mid to late 1990's.(56) This is incredibly alarming. (Not only is this devastating for these children and for their families, but the long term societal consequences are of major concern as well. Here are a few of the long term concerns according to the organization Autism Speaks(2):

On average, autism costs an estimated $60,000 a year through childhood, with the bulk of the costs in special services and lost wages related to increased demands on one or both parents. Costs increase with the occurrence of intellectual disability.

Mothers of children with ASD, who tend to serve as the child's case manager and advocate, are less likely to work outside the home. On average, they work fewer hours per week and earn 56 percent less than mothers of children with no health limitations and 35 percent less than mothers of children with other disabilities or disorders.

Over the next decade, an estimated 707,000 to 1,116,000 teens (70,700 to 111,600 each year) will enter adulthood and age out of school based autism services.

More than half of young adults with autism remain unemployed and unenrolled in higher education in the two years after high school. This is a lower rate than that of young adults in other disability categories, including learning disabilities, intellectual disability or speech-language impairment.

Of the nearly 18,000 people with autism who used state-funded vocational rehabilitation programs in 2014, only 60 percent left the program with a job. Of these, 80 percent worked part-time at a median weekly rate of $160, putting them well below the poverty level.

The cost of caring for Americans with autism had reached $268 billion in 2015 and would rise to $461 billion by 2025 in the absence of more-effective interventions and support across the life span.

The majority of autism's costs in the U.S. are for adult services – an estimated $175 to $196 billion a year, compared to $61 to $66 billion a year for children.

- On average, medical expenditures for children and adolescents with ASD were 4.1 to 6.2 times greater than for those without autism.

As you can see, this is an issue with enormous problems for the families affected and for everyone in our society. This is an issue that can not be ignored and will not simply go away. Just for the record, Autism Speaks states on their web page that the "results of research are clear, vaccines do not cause autism." This is what they have been told by the higher powers that they trust (so they are simply following the script). As you are about to see however, this is not reality.

Found in the Congressional Record from May 21, 2003, there are many highly accredited doctors who seem to also think that this topic is far from settled. Dr. Boyd E. Haley, who is the Chairman of the Chemistry Department at the University of Kentucky summarized his views in this way: "I cannot say, nor would I say, that vaccinations cause autism. However, if the data holds up that I have been seeing with the relationship, I think it is an awfully good suspect, at least one of the co-factors that might aid in the onset of this disease. We clearly know infants' brains are more sensitive. We know the blood-brain barrier, the barrier to drugs between the blood and the brain, is virtually gone in infants. At the recent International Meeting for Autism Research at the Society for Neuroscience, a number of investigators around the world are finding similar things. At Columbia University, there's now a model in mice who were injected with low doses of thimerosal very similar to what's given in human vaccines. These mice develop neurological deficits that look like autism, and when you take their brains out and you analyze them, they have the same type of brain damage."(1) One of my favorite parts of this statement is when Dr. Haley says that vaccines could be "at least one of the co-factors that might aid in the onset of this disease." He is intelligent enough to see the plausibility and not dismiss the possibility that vaccines may (at the very least) be a part of the problem. And for the record, health freedom advocates are not suggesting that vaccines are the only cause or reason for autism either.

Another prominent doctor who testified in the Congressional record in 2003 was Dr. Thomas Verstraeten, formerly of the EIS office at the National Immunization Program, who utilized the Vaccine Safety Datalink to evaluate any possible connection between thimerosal-preserved vaccines and neurological or renal impairment. He found, "a statistically significant positive correlation between the cumulative exposure at 2 months and unspecified developmental delay; the cumulative exposure at 3 months and tics; the cumulative exposure at 6 months and attention deficit disorder . . . 1, 3 and 6 months and language and speech delay . . . 1, 3, and 6 months of age and neurodevelopmental delays in general." He concludes: "This analysis suggests that in our study population, the risks of tics, ADD, language and speech delays, and developmental delays in general may be increased by exposures to mercury from thimerosal-containing vaccines during the first six months of life."(1) An interesting thing is that one of the studies most often quoted by those saying that the science proves that vaccines do not cause autism is one completed by Dr. Verstraeten. (3) An even more interesting thing regarding this particular study that the proponents of vaccines love to quote, is that the good doctor wrote a rather irate letter to the editor of the journal *Pediatrics* which published his study. In his letter he expressed his concern that the journal had mis-represented his study by stating that the study proved there was no link between vaccines and autism. "The article does not state that we found evidence against an association, as a negative study would. It does state, on the contrary, that additional study is recommended, which is the conclusion to which a neutral study must come. A neutral study carries a very distinct message: the investigators could neither confirm nor exclude an association, and therefore more study is required."(4) Dr. Verstraeten was quoted again in the Congressional document as saying, "Unfortunately I have witnessed how many experts, looking at this thimerosal issue, do not seem bothered to compare apples to pears and insist if nothing is happening in these studies, then nothing should be feared of thimerosal. I do not wish to be the advocate of the anti-vaccine lobby and sound as if I am convinced that thimerosal is or was harmful; but at least I feel we should use sound scientific argumentation, and not let our standards be dictated by our desire to disprove an unpleasant theory."(1) Similar to

Dr. Haley, Dr. Verstraeten seems to see the distinct possibility of a connection and as a scientist does not want anyone to simply dismiss the role that vaccines may play.

Two more medical doctors quoted in the Congressional document Dr. David Baskin and Dr. George Lucier discussed the dangers of thimerosal. Dr. David Baskin, M.D., professor of neurological surgery, Baylor College of Medicine, stated, "There is more data, more and more data on ethylmercury (thimerosal). The cells that I showed you dying in cell culture are dying from ethylmercury. Those are human frontal brain cells." Dr. George Lucier, the former Director of the Environmental Toxicology Program at the National Institutes of Health, stated, "Ethylmercury is a neurotoxin. Infants may be more susceptible than adults."(1) Contrary to the blanket statements that the vaccine apologists continue making regarding the safety of vaccines, not everyone agrees with their conclusion that thimerosal is harmless, nor do they seem to agree that there is "no connection between vaccines and autism."

The Congressional record also shows very real concern that the vaccine-autism connection was not being taken seriously by some of the government agencies and their researchers, "Of additional concern has been the CDC's bias against theories regarding vaccine-induced autism. Rather than aggressively work to replicate clinical findings with laboratory data that showed a relationship between vaccines and autism, the CDC funded researchers who also worked for vaccine manufacturers to conduct population-based epidemiological studies to look at the possible correlation between vaccine injury and a subset of the population that might be injured."(1) Chairman Burton went further in expressing some of his concerns: "Officials at HHS have aggressively denied any possible connection between vaccines and autism. They have waged an information campaign endorsing one conclusion on an issue where the science is still out."(1)

At the beginning of this chapter I showed a quote from the CDC which stated that, "Vaccines do not cause autism." "Vaccine ingredients do not cause autism." The CDC uses one major study to use as their proof for those statements and that is the IOM reports. In the reports the IOM states, "The evidence favors rejection of a causal relationship at the population level between MMR vaccine and autism spectrum disorders." Of course this is where the CDC leaves things because by doing so it makes it seem as though the IOM report is proving what they so fervently wish for. However, if we continue with the IOM's report...they found insufficient evidence to accept or reject a connection between thimerosal in vaccines and autism. They did, however, state that such a connection is "biologically plausible," and recommended much more research on the issue. "The committee concludes that the evidence is inadequate to accept or reject a causal relationship between exposure to thimerosal from vaccines and the neurodevelopmental disorders of autism, ADHD, and speech or language delay."(1) This report has been used like a hammer to beat the "vaccines do not cause autism" script into the minds of those that will listen. The IOM report clearly states that there was not enough information/evidence to make a conclusion. They also clearly stated that more evidence was necessary and that the connection was "biologically plausible." Yet this is not how the reported information is being disseminated to the media or public. There is another statement that tends to circulate among the defenders of the vaccine story line, "the science is settled." Probably one of the most vile statements to my ears, as the entire idea that science is settled goes against everything that defines actual science. By utilizing this erroneous statement as some kind of factual statement, they are attempting to keep individuals from accepting any research other than what they deem to be acceptable. Because, of course, if the science is actually settled then why should we be listening to anyone telling us otherwise.

The following are all studies that show some correlation between vaccines and autism. The vaccine apologists have their handful of studies that they will pull out to try and convince the public that the science is settled and to try to make their case stronger they will attempt to discredit all of these studies listed here as somehow being inadequate and inferior to anything they have produced. Yet notice that different researchers from all over the world are coming to many of the same conclusions...that there is a correlation between vaccines and autism. As an aside, there are plenty of individuals who have dissected the studies that supposedly prove that vaccines do not cause autism and the fact that there is plenty to be dissected in these studies that never gets discussed in the media clearly shows the script at work. (5,6,7) Yet another interesting tidbit to consider is that Poul Thorsen, one of the primary researchers responsible for producing the major studies that supposedly prove the no-autism-link opinion has been on the FBI most wanted list since 2012. He was placed on this list because he was indicted on 22 counts of fraud. This fraud is based on schemes to steal money from the CDC through grant money ear-marked for autism research. So please, take your time with the following list so that you can see for yourself that the science is far from settled. For the record this is a highly abbreviated list of what is out there showing all of the possible links between vaccines and autism.

1. "Serological association of measles virus and human herpesvirus-6 with brain autoantibodies in autism." "This study is the first to report an association between virus serology and brain autoantibody in autism; it supports the hypothesis that a virus-induced autoimmune response may play a causal role in autism."(8)

2. "Administration of thimerosal to infant rats increases overflow of glutamate and aspartate in the prefrontal cortex: protective role of dehydroepiandrosterone sulfate." "Since excessive accumulation of extracellular glutamate is linked with excitotoxicity, our data imply that neonatal exposure to thimerosal-containing vaccines might induce excitotoxic brain injuries, leading to neurodevelopmental disorders."(9)

3. "B-lymphocytes from a population of children with autism spectrum disorder and their unaffected siblings exhibit hypersensitivity to thimerosal." "Cells hypersensitive to thimerosal also had higher levels of oxidative stress markers, protein carbonyls, and oxidant generation. This suggests certain individuals with a mild mitochondrial defect may be highly susceptible to mitochondrial specific toxins like the vaccine preservative thimerosal." (10)

4. “Risk factors for autistic regression: results of an ambispective cohort study.” “This study suggests that febrile seizures (a known adverse vaccine event) and family history of neuropsychiatric disorders are correlated with autistic regression.” (11)

5. “Persistent behavioral impairments and alterations of brain dopamine system after early postnatal administration of thimerosal in rats.” “These data document that early postnatal THIM (thimerosal) administration causes lasting neurobehavioral impairments and neurochemical alterations in the brain, dependent on dose and sex. If similar changes occur in THIM/mercurial-exposed children, they could contribute to neurodevelopmental disorders.” (12)

6. “Do aluminum vaccine adjuvants contribute to the rising prevalence of autism?” “We show that Al(aluminum)-adjuvanted vaccines may be a significant etiological factor in the rising prevalence of ASD in the Western world. We also show that children from countries with the highest ASD prevalence appear to have a much higher exposure to Al from vaccines, particularly at 2 months of age.”(13)

7. “Possible immunological disorders in autism: concomitant autoimmunity and immune tolerance.” “It is concluded that autoimmune response to dietary proteins and deficient immune response to measles, mumps and rubella vaccine antigens might be associated with autism, as a leading cause or a resulting event.”(14)

8. “A case series of children with apparent mercury toxic encephalopathies manifesting with clinical symptoms of regressive autistic disorders.” “Evidence for mercury intoxication should be considered in the differential diagnosis as contributing to some regressive ASDs.”(15)

9. “A positive association found between autism prevalence and childhood vaccination uptake across the U.S. population.” “The results suggest that although mercury has been removed from many vaccines, other culprits may link vaccines to autism. Further study into the relationship between vaccines and autism is warranted.” (16)

10. “Induction of metallothionein in mouse cerebellum and cerebrum with low-dose thimerosal injection.” “The results support the hy-

pothesis that Hg (mercury) sensitivity may be a heritable/genetic risk factor for ASD."(17)

11. "Abnormal measles-mumps-rubella antibodies and CNS autoimmunity in children with autism." "Stemming from this evidence, we suggest that an inappropriate antibody response to MMR, specifically the measles component thereof, might be related to pathogenesis of autism."(18)

12. "Influence of pediatric vaccines on amygdala growth and opioid ligand binding in rhesus macaque infants: A pilot study." "These results suggest that maturational changes in amygdala volume and the binding capacity of [11C]DPN in the amygdala was significantly altered in infant macaques receiving the vaccine schedule."(19)

13. "Lasting neuropathological changes in rat brain after intermittent neonatal administration of thimerosal." "These findings document neurotoxic effects of thimerosal, at doses equivalent to those used in infant vaccines or higher, in developing rat brain, suggesting likely involvement of this mercurial in neurodevelopmental disorders."(20)

14. "A Cross-Sectional Study of the Association between Infant Hepatitis B Vaccine Exposure in Boys and the Risk of Adverse Effects as Measured by Receipt of Special Education Services." "This study supports a significant about nine-fold increase in the risk of adverse effects as measured by receipt of special education services among boys receiving infant Thimerosal-containing hepatitis B vaccination."(21)

15. "Hepatitis B triple series vaccine and developmental disability in US children aged 1–9 years." "This study found statistically significant evidence to suggest that boys in United States who were vaccinated with the triple series Hepatitis B vaccine, during the time period in which vaccines were manufactured with thimerosal, were more susceptible to developmental disability than were unvaccinated boys."(22)

16. "Neurotoxic effects of postnatal thimerosal are mouse strain dependent." "These findings implicate genetic influences and provide a model for investigating thimerosal-related neurotoxicity."(23)

17. "Detection of Measles Virus Genomic RNA in Cerebrospinal Fluid of Children with Regressive Autism." "This study reports for the first time simultaneous detection of MV genomic RNA in at least two sites–ileal lymphoid tissue and CSF–in three children with regressive autism."(24)

18. "A positive association found between autism prevalence and childhood vaccination uptake across the U.S. population." "The results suggest that although mercury has been removed from many vaccines, other culprits may link vaccines to autism. Further study into the relationship between vaccines and autism is warranted."(25)

19. "Immunological findings in autism." "Mercury and an infectious agent like the measles virus are currently two main candidate environmental triggers for immune dysfunction in autism. The possibility of its involvement in autism cannot be ruled out."(26)

20. "Focal brain inflammation and autism." "Increasing evidence indicates that brain inflammation is important in the pathogenesis of neuropsychiatric disorders"(27)

21. "Neuroglial activation and neuroinflammation in the brain of patients with autism." "We demonstrate an active neuroinflammatory process in the cerebral cortex, white matter, and notably in cerebellum of autistic patients."(28)

22. "Inflammation and Neuro-Immune Dysregulations in Autism Spectrum Disorders." "Neuro-inflammation and neuro-immune abnormalities have now been established in ASD development and maintenance."(29)

23. "B-Lymphocytes from a Population of Children with Autism Spectrum Disorder and Their Unaffected Siblings Exhibit Hypersensitivity to Thimerosal." "This suggests certain individuals with a mild mitochondrial defect may be highly susceptible to mitochondrial specific toxins like the vaccine preservative thimerosal."(30)

24. "A case series of children with apparent mercury toxic encephalopathies manifesting with clinical symptoms of regressive autistic disorders." "Evidence for mercury intoxication should be consid-

ered in the differential diagnosis as contributing to some regressive ASDs."(31)

25. "An evaluation of the effects of thimerosal on neurodevelopmental disorders reported following DTP and Hib vaccines in comparison to DTPH vaccine in the United States." "Significantly increased odds ratios for autism, speech disorders, mental retardation, infantile spasms, and thinking abnormalities reported to VAERS were found following DTP vaccines in comparison to DTPH vaccines with minimal bias or systematic error."(32)

26. "Hepatitis B vaccination of male neonates and autism diagnosis, NHIS 1997-2002." "Findings suggest that U.S. male neonates vaccinated with the hepatitis B vaccine prior to 1999 (from vaccination record) had a threefold higher risk for parental report of autism diagnosis compared to boys not vaccinated as neonates during that same time period. Nonwhite boys bore a greater risk."(33)

27. "Neurodevelopmental disorders, maternal Rh-negativity, and Rho(D) immune globulins: a multi-center assessment." "This study associates TCR exposure with some NDs in children."(34)

28. "A positive association found between autism prevalence and childhood vaccination uptake across the U.S. population." "The results suggest that although mercury has been removed from many vaccines, other culprits may link vaccines to autism. Further study into the relationship between vaccines and autism is warranted."(35)

29. "Thimerosal Exposure and the Role of Sulfation Chemistry and Thiol Availability in Autism." "Research indicates that the availability of thiols, particularly GSH, can influence the effects of thimerosal (TM) and other mercury (Hg) compounds."(36)

30. "Thimerosal exposure in infants and neurodevelopmental disorders: an assessment of computerized medical records in the Vaccine Safety Datalink." "Consistent significantly increased rate ratios were observed for autism, autism spectrum disorders, tics, attention deficit disorder, and emotional disturbances with Hg exposure from TCVs."(37)

31. "Thimerosal-Derived Ethylmercury Is a Mitochondrial Toxin in Human Astrocytes: Possible Role of Fenton Chemistry in the Oxidation and Breakage of mtDNA." "The results of this study suggest that ethylmercury is a mitochondrial toxin in human astrocytes."(38)

32. "Thimerosal induces neuronal cell apoptosis by causing cytochrome c and apoptosis-inducing factor release from mitochondria." "In this study, we show that thimerosal, at nanomolar concentrations, induces neuronal cell death through the mitochondrial pathway."(39)

32. "Aluminum in brain tissue in autism." "The pre-eminence of intracellular aluminum associated with non-neuronal cells was a standout observation in autism brain tissue and may offer clues as to both the origin of the brain aluminum as well as a putative role in autism spectrum disorder." (40)

32. "Reconsideration of the immunotherapeutic pediatric safe dose levels of aluminum." "Our calculations show that the levels of aluminum suggested by the currently used limits place infants at risk of acute, repeated, and possibly chronic exposures of toxic levels of aluminum in modern vaccine schedules."(41)

So let's look again at the script the vaccine apologists love to use.(42)

The Centers for Disease Control and Prevention (CDC)
"Many studies have looked at whether there is a relationship between vaccines and autism. The weight of the evidence indicates that vaccines are not associated with autism."

The National Institutes of Health (NIH)
"There is no conclusive evidence that any part of a vaccine or combination of vaccines causes autism, even though researchers have done many studies to answer this important question. There is also no proof that any material used to make or preserve the vaccine plays a role in causing autism. Although there have been reports of studies that relate vaccines to autism, these findings have not held up under further investigation."

American Academy of Pediatrics (AAP)
"Scientific data does not show a link between vaccines and autism."

Their statements make me think of a quote which is from one of my favorite movies, The Princess Bride, "Why do you keep using that word, I do not think it means what you think it means." They are like a broken record. Again, let me remind you that although their statements do not clarify it, these statements are really only making observations regarding the MMR vaccine and more specifically the one ingredient, thimerosal.

On August 27, 2014, William Thompson, PhD., a long time senior scientist with the CDC, became a whistleblower. The following statement is taken directly from the press release that was given out by his lawyers back in 2014: "I regret that my co-authors and I omitted statistically significant information in our 2004 article published in the journal Pediatrics (this paper has been widely used to support the script of vaccines do not cause autism). The omitted data suggested that African American males who received the MMR vaccine before age 36 months were at increased risk for autism. Decisions were made regarding which findings to report after the data were collected, and I believe that the final study protocol was not followed. I want to be absolutely clear that I believe vaccines have saved and continue to save countless lives."(43) Dr. Thompson stated that the changes that were made to the final study would have shown a significant risk of autism, especially in African American boys. "The omitted data suggested that African-American males who received the MMR vaccine before age 36 months were at increased risk for autism. Decisions were made regarding which findings to report after the data were collected, and I believe that the final study protocol was not followed."(44) As is the usual result, any time something becomes public that sheds any ill light upon vaccines it is immediately set upon by the vaccine defenders. The information is explained as false or misleading and the persons involved are systematically destroyed and discredited.

Dr. Thompson had two other studies in which links to thimerosal vaccines and tics in boys were shown.(45)(46) Tics are a common finding in some of the research listed in this chapter. According to Dr. Thompson, different officials within the CDC pressured him to downplay the relationships between the vaccines and the tics in young boys.(47) Dr. Thompson stated that, "tics were like five times more common in children with autism."(47) One of the criticisms that the apologists like to bring up is that to date Dr. Thompson has remained silent. The reality behind that criticism is that Dr. Thompson still works for the CDC and "according to the Whistle Blower Protection Act and other federal regulations, Dr. Thompson can not testify under oath without the permission of the director of the CDC, Dr. Thomas Frieden."(47) However, that request for his testimonial has been denied. "In denying the request, Dr. Frieden said, "Dr. William Thompson's deposition testimony would not substantially promote the objectives of CDC or HHS [Health and Human Services]."(47)

The vaccine apologists attempt to make out Dr. Thompson as some lone rogue doctor whose information was never verified. To give some further context to his allegations you would need to be aware of other whistleblowers. In 2016, a group calling themselves SPIDER (Scientists Preserving Integrity, Diligence and Ethics in Research), "put a list of complaints in writing in a letter to CDC Chief of Staff and provided a copy of the letter to the public watchdog organization U.S. Right to Know (USRTK). The members of the group have elected to file the complaint anonymously for fear of retribution."(48) In the letter they declared that, "It appears that our mission is being influenced and shaped by outside parties and rogue interests… and Congressional intent for our agency is being circumvented by some of our leaders. What concerns us most, is that it is becoming the norm and not the rare exception," the letter states. "These questionable and unethical practices threaten to undermine our credibility and reputation as a trusted leader in public health."(48) Among their accusations against the CDC was this one that relates directly to Dr. Thompson's own accusations, "Definitions were changed and data 'cooked' to make the results look better than they were," the complaint states. "An 'internal review' that involved staff across CDC occurred and its findings were essentially suppressed so media and/or Congressional staff would not become aware of the problems."(48) Another incident that also relates directly to Dr. Thompson's allegations occurred back in 2010, "Stephen A. Krahling and Joan A. Wlochowski, former Merck virologists blew the whistle by filing a qui tam action lawsuit (U.S. v

Merck & Co.) The suit charges that Merck knew its measles, mumps, rubella (MMR) vaccine was less effective than the purported 95% level, and it alleges that senior management was aware and also oversaw testing that concealed the actual effectiveness. According to the lawsuit, Merck began a sham testing program in the late 1990's to hide the declining efficacy of the vaccine. The objective of the fraudulent trials was to "report efficacy of 95% or higher regardless of the vaccine's true efficacy."(49) They went on to say that "they were threatened with jail were they to alert the FDA to the fraud being committed."(49)

I am well aware that neither of these other whistleblowing reports proves Dr. Thompson was telling the truth. However, the corroborating accounts of cover up and fraud should at least give him some credence that he is possibly telling the truth. In Point Number 4, Trust for a Liability Free Product, I gave you dozens of examples of lawsuits against pharmaceutical companies that contain numerous examples of fraud. To understand all of this information and still walk away thinking there is no way the CDC would have lied (or is still lying) about the link between vaccines and autism is to be trusting beyond all comprehension.

One other point I would like to show here to increase your understanding about how there absolutely could be a link between vaccines and autism and how researchers should be digging harder to find the link instead of simply trying to disprove a negative. This last point has to do with brain inflammation and vaccines. Encephalopathy (a disease in which the functioning of the brain is affected by some agent or condition) and encephalitis (inflammation of the active tissues of the brain caused by an infection or an autoimmune response) are both recognized in the Vaccine Injury Table as being able to be caused by vaccines. There have also been numerous research papers that discuss this: "Post-vaccination Acute disseminated encephalomyelitis (ADEM) has been associated with several vaccines such as rabies, diphtheria-tetanus-polio, smallpox, measles, mumps, rubella, Japanese B encephalitis, pertussis, influenza, hepatitis B, and the Hog vaccine."(50) "A total of 48 children, ages 10 to 49 months, met the inclusion criteria after receiving measles vaccine, alone or in combination. Eight children died, and the remainder had mental regression and retardation, chronic seizures, motor and sensory deficits, and movement disorders. This clustering suggests that a causal relationship between measles vaccine and encephalopathy may exist as a rare complication of measles immunization."(51) Brain inflammation is also a component of autism.(27)(28)(29) At least one study speaks directly to the relationship between vaccine induced encephalopathy and autism, "these previously normally developing children suffered mercury toxic encephalopathies that manifested with clinical symptoms consistent with regressive ASDs."(15) Another research paper discusses inflammation that is caused by the adjuvants found in vaccines (not just the thimerosal), ""The autoimmune/inflammatory syndrome induced by adjuvants (ASIA) is a recently identified condition in which the exposure to an adjuvant leads to an aberrant autoimmune response."(52) When you look at some of the characteristics of encephalopathy/ encephalitis things get very interesting: an altered mental state, loss of memory and cognitive ability, subtle personality changes, inability to concentrate, lethargy, progressive loss of consciousness, seizures, loss of ability to swallow or speak, muscle atrophy and weakness.(53) Compare this list to the characteristics found in autism and you may be shocked. The ability to differentiate between these characteristics and then be able to assert with complete confidence that vaccines do not cause autism and even more bold to say that there is absolutely no link between the two, is absurd. In fact that is exactly what a paper written by Pace Environmental Law Review stated, "Based on this preliminary assessment, there may be no meaningful distinction between the cases of encephalopathy and residual seizure disorder that the VICP compensated over the last twenty years and the cases of "autism" that the VICP has denied."(54) In a "learning module (that) was developed based on a needs survey sent to all third year medicine clerkship directors and all medicine residency program directors in the United States." The FDA clearly points out to all of these medical professionals how determining adverse drug reactions (ADR) should take place. "It can be hard to determine if an individual drug caused a reaction in a complicated patient receiving multiple medications. However, the temporal relationship of a reaction with regard to the administration of a new medication can be helpful. Also, biological plausibility (asking if the drug's mechanism of action makes this possible or likely) can also be helpful. The bottom line is, even when in doubt about whether a drug caused the reaction, report it." Temporal relationship and biological plausibility, the two things pointed out here in this presentation meant to train medical professionals how to look for ADRs are the exact two things we are told to ignore when it comes to vaccines.(55)

In an excellent book titled *The Environmental and Genetic Causes of Autism*, James Lyons-Weiler, PHD gives a multitude of highly plausible and well researched hypotheses for a connection between vaccines and autism. In this book Lyons-Weiler states that the CDC, "seem to not be aware or to care about the science showing other compounds and exposures that might lead to autism via microglial activation, such as the science showing that glyphosate may be a causal factor and acetaminophen/ASD links. They are asleep at the wheel on these other important factors, but they are actively misleading the public on vaccine safety." His book is a must read for anyone who truly wants to understand the intricacies involved in the autism epidemic. A separate paper written by Lyons-Weiler in the academic journal, *Autism-Open Access* in 2018 continued the discussion created in his book and adds to the original ideas further reinforcing the model that he has created for looking into the causes of autism. (56) The image below is a visual for his ASD causality model.

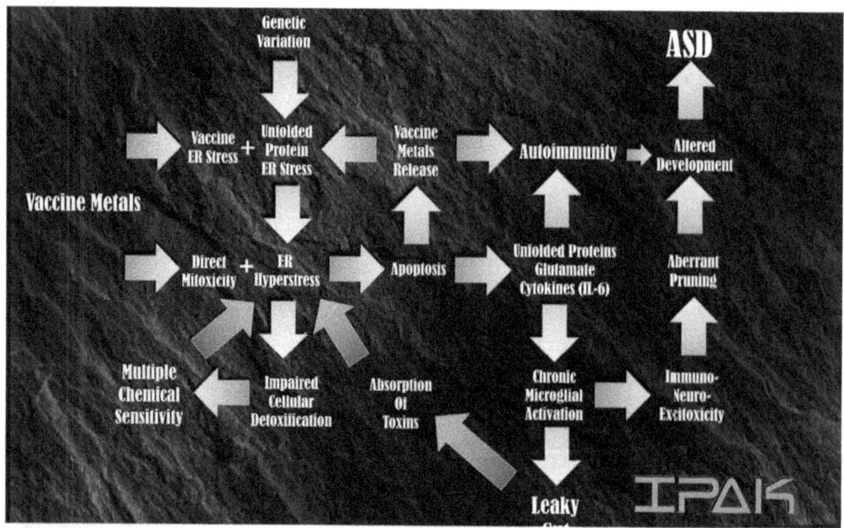

For decades government lawyers have used medical experts in trials to insist that there is no connection between vaccines and autism. These experts talk about encephalopathy and autism like there could in no way be any link or commonality. That is until one of their experts changed their tune. Dr. Andrew Zimmerman is a pediatric neurologist with a very long list of accolades who was used as one of these expert witnesses for the government. He testified numerous times that vaccines do not cause autism in specific patients. However when the good doctor had a change of opinion based on seeing new evidence and informed the government that vaccines could cause autism in "exceptional" cases, he states that the government hid the information and misrepresented his opinion. He, of course, was promptly fired as an expert witness for the government. I wonder how many more doctors like Dr. Zimmerman there are out there who had a similar experience with our government? (57)

Probably the most common statement made in regard to this issue is that correlation does not equal causation. Of course this is an accurate statement in any scenario. Just because there is correlation, and no matter how much correlation exists, it still does not lead directly to causation. There can still be confounding factors, a directionality issue or simply coincidence. One way of establishing causation (as mentioned previously) is through temporal precedence, meaning that the "hypothesized cause comes before the measured effect." (58) In thousands of separate and individual interviews with parents of autistic children, the one common denominator they all had was that their child was labeled as healthy or thriving by their pediatrician and then within 24-48 hours after a vaccination the child began to deteriorate or regress. The thousands of parents are then told that this is merely coincidence. Unfortunately, temporal precedence is not enough to establish the cause of autism. This is where the appropriate testing must come in. The vaccine apologists will say that the subject of vaccines and autism is a closed book, however they say this without actually having done the appropriate science to make this claim. The lack of large-scale, unbiased studies leaves very critical questions completely unanswered. The databases are available to look at this subject more rigorously but they are not being utilized. Ignoring these issues highlights a flawed system that prioritizes narrative over scientific exploration.

Finally, I want to bring up the Hannah Poling case. The vaccine defenders love to say that vaccines do not cause autism and they love to shout to the heavens that no evidence exists to prove otherwise. When this particular case is brought up they like to say that it did not prove anything. Well, I beg to differ. Hannah's case was one of six cases used in the Omnibus Autism Proceedings, which was a kind of kangaroo court set up to prove that there was no link between vaccines and autism. Six cases were hand selected to represent more than 5,000 pending vaccine-autism cases and the goal was to prove these cases false so that they could then deny all of the other pending cases. This was their goal. During these proceedings, they decided against 5 of the 6 cases (and the information behind these cases is very shifty), however they quietly settled, then sealed Hannah's case. Bottom line, she was awarded nearly 20 million over her lifetime because...wait for it...vaccines were found to have been a causative agent in her autism. It was only after this information was leaked to the press that we discovered it.(59)

Why does our government insist on the continuing script that there is absolutely no evidence, no link, no correlation at all between vaccines and autism? Why? How about to avoid paying potentially trillions in compensation ordered by Congress. That is the possible cost to our government to pay out to all of the millions of children and their families who have been harmed through this cover up. The cost to those responsible behind the campaign of deceit and lies both financially, legally and the failure of all trust is what motivates them to continue fighting a smear campaign against anyone who speaks out against vaccines. As was stated in the article regarding the Hannah Poling case, "Paying claims to all those children with autism would quickly bankrupt the program..." No matter how much evidence, no matter how much logic, no matter how much testimony to the truth they just keep on fighting. They continue to turn their collective blind-eye to the thousands of families who repeat nearly identical stories of how their children were documented by their pediatricians as progressing perfectly normal right up to the point they declined into autism after being injected with vaccines. They continue to slander highly respected and credentialed scientists and doctors who show any sign of going against their script. But the truth can not be silenced. In the end it is the truth that shall prevail.

Point Number Nine
Vaccinated versus unvaccinated

"To find the truth, you must first be willing to question everything."
~Anonymous

If you want to get the correct answer to a question when doing research it is paramount that you compare and contrast the right things. If you are really wanting to know if the drug that you created is causing a serious issue then it would make sense to set up an experiment that would clearly illustrate whether or not the drug is the cause of this issue, right? Let's say I have a drug that is supposed to help people with chronic migraines. Now suppose there is a question as to whether the drug may be causing a serious side effect. To find out if it is true, one of the easiest ways would be to create an experiment and give the drug to one large group of people and not give the drug to another large group of people. Did the group that got the drug have this serious side effect? Did the one that did not receive the drug get the serious side effect? If the group that took the drug had a statistically significant higher number of people with this side effect then we have a winner, or loser depending on how you look at it. But of course that is only what you would do if you actually wanted to find the answer to the question.

In the world of vaccines and their side effects, the questions are numerous. Does vaccination cause autism? Does vaccination cause an increase in allergies? How about asthma? Arthritis? Guillain-Barre Syndrome? How about autoimmune issues? What are the long term adverse effects from having multiple vaccinations? The questions go on and on. So we pick one at random...allergies. Now if the powers that be actually want to know the answer to whether or not vaccination can increase the risk of allergic reactions in a population they would need to create a study that contains a large group of children receiving vaccines and compare them to a large group of children who are not receiving the vaccines. We would then need to follow these groups for a significant length of time to be able to observe what happens. Then at the end of the study we should be able to clearly see if one group did better than the other. This should easily give us the answer we are looking for, right? Theoretically. Would it surprise you to know that neither the pharmaceutical companies nor the CDC have ever done any large, long-term studies comparing the long-term health of fully vaccinated individuals versus those who have never been vaccinated to try and seek out any of these answers? It's true, this has never been done. Ever! Like I said, you have to want to know the answers.

With that said, this does not mean that there are no studies that compare vaccinated and unvaccinated individuals. There are in fact quite a few of those to be found and with some very interesting results as well. As we do not have a large, long-term study to compare the long-term health of those that have been fully vaccinated to those who have never been vaccinated we must attempt to extrapolate information from the studies that we do have. This is a poor alternative and does not give us the information that we truly need in order to find the links to the myriad of issues that may be stemming from vaccines. If finding an answer were actually what the vaccine apologists really wanted then creating a study as mentioned would not be an entirely difficult process to set up. There are numerous families, and for that matter, entire groups of people, that have chosen to not vaccinate their children. If asked, I have no doubt that they would be more than willing to participate in some type of long-term study to look at the differences between their (100%) unvaccinated children and the other (100%) vaccinated children.

The vaccine apologists will argue that any long-term study that denies any group of children a vaccine is unethical and immoral.(1) The idea being that vaccines are a proven entity and as such this means that if we deny them to children in a study it is unethical and immoral.

It is an entirely convenient theory for them to fall back on and deny their ability to perform the necessary research. Finding families who would sign off on a study as is being suggested should not be that difficult. This should mitigate the excuse of unethical and immoral reasons for not performing said study. The vaccine apologists know this. This is a topic that has been brought forward to various groups and panels over the past several decades and each and every time the end result is that nothing happens. So understanding that we may never see a proper long-term study to look at the differences between (100%) unvaccinated children and (100%) vaccinated children, let's at least look at the studies that we can look at.

Let's look at some of what we do have available and see if we can extrapolate some answers from the information gained from these studies.

In a study designed to investigate the association between vaccination with the Hepatitis B triple series vaccine prior to 2000 and developmental disability in children aged 1–9 years, the authors of this first study we are looking at found that the "odds of receiving EIS (Early Intervention Services) were approximately nine times as great for vaccinated boys (n = 46) as for unvaccinated boys (n = 7), after adjustment for confounders." They concluded that the "study found statistically significant evidence to suggest that boys in the United States who were vaccinated with the triple series Hepatitis B vaccine, during the time period in which vaccines were manufactured with thimerosal, were more susceptible to developmental disability than were unvaccinated boys."(2)

In this next study, by the same authors of the previous study, they wished to go a step further than their last study and try to see if there was an increased risk of autism with the hepatitis B vaccine. Their findings "suggest that U.S. male neonates vaccinated with the hepatitis B vaccine prior to 1999 (from vaccination record) had a threefold higher risk for parental report of autism diagnosis compared to boys not vaccinated as neonates during that same time period. Nonwhite boys bore a greater risk."(3) As you may remember from Point 8, that last bit of information is the same finding that the infamous Thompson study on autism found (and was covered up).(4)

In another study that was done on the HPV vaccine, they utilized a questionnaire form with 275 questions that were answered from 30,793 respondents. Of those, 21,034 were vaccinated, 9,245 unvaccinated and 514 were unclear. "By using binary answers ("yes"/"no") for the question on individual HPV vaccine administration, the respondents were categorized into the "vaccinated case" group or the "unvaccinated control" group." Their "analyses demonstrated that the vaccinated cases were significantly more likely than unvaccinated controls to have experienced symptoms of memory impairment and involuntary movement."(5)

This next study looked only at whether or not a group had been vaccinated with DTP or not vaccinated with DTP, so it was not a true vaccinated/unvaccinated study. It was simply looking at whether an individual had received this one particular vaccine or not. "The odds of having a history of asthma was twice as great among vaccinated subjects than among unvaccinated subjects (adjusted odds ratio, 2.00). The odds of having had any allergy-related respiratory symptom in the past 12 months was 63% greater among vaccinated subjects than unvaccinated subjects. DTP or tetanus vaccination appears to increase the risk of allergies and related respiratory symptoms in children and adolescents."(6)

In another study involving the DTP vaccine, the authors "compared 3–5-month-old children who had received DTP (± Oral Polio Vaccine) vaccinations early with children who had not yet received these vaccinations. When unvaccinated controls were normal children who had not yet been eligible for vaccination, mortality was 5 times higher for DTP-vaccinated children. The estimated effects of DTP and OPV are unlikely to have been influenced by other vaccinations since very few had received other vaccines; if the children who may have received BCG (Bacillus Calmette–Guérin vaccine is a vaccine primarily used against tuberculosis) were censored in the analysis the result was essentially the same."(7)

In the following study, the researchers set out "to examine the risk of neurological and autoimmune disorders of special interest in people vaccinated against pandemic influenza A (H1N1) with Pandemrix compared with unvaccinated people over 8-10 months," the authors found that "relative risks were significantly increased for Bell's palsy, paraesthesia, and inflammatory bowel disease after vaccination, predominantly in the early phase of the vaccination campaign." This study looked at a large number of individuals to come to that conclusion, "All people registered in Stockholm county on 1 October 2009 and who had lived in this region since 1 January 1998; 1,024,019 were vaccinated against H1N1 and 921,005 remained unvaccinated."(8)

This next study is very interesting for several reasons. This was an unpublished CDC study discovered through a Freedom of Information Act (FOIA) request, authors Versraeten and DeStefano (the Director of the Immunization Safety office at the CDC) found that the "relative risk (RR) of developing a neurologic development disorder was 1.8 (80% higher) when comparing the highest exposure group at 1 month of age to the unexposed group. "Within this group we also found an elevated risk for the following disorders: autism (RR 7.6), nonorganic sleep disorders (RR 5.0), and speech disorders (RR 2.1). This analysis suggests that high exposure to ethylmercury from thimerosal-containing vaccines in the first month of life increases the risk of subsequent development of neurologic development impairment." It is not specified whether the "unexposed" group had received other vaccines that did not contain thimerosal.(9)

And finally we have four studies that probably come the closest to the (100%) vaccinated versus (100%) unvaccinated study that we have been wanting for so long. Each of these studies compares groups of children who were either fully vaccinated or unvaccinated (sometimes a third group of partially vaccinated) and looks for long-term health consequences.

The lead author on this first study was Anthony R. Mawson, Professor, Department of Epidemiology and Biostatistics, School of Public Health, Jackson State University. "The information contained in 415 questionnaires provided data on 666 homeschool children. With regard to vaccination status, 261 (39%) were unvaccinated, 208 (31%) were partially vaccinated, and 197 (30%) had received all of the recommended vaccinations. Vaccinated children were significantly more likely than the unvaccinated to have been diagnosed with the following: allergic rhinitis (10.4% vs. 0.4%), other allergies (22.2% vs. 6.9%), eczema/ atopic dermatitis (9.5% vs. 3.6%), a learning disability (5.7% vs. 1.2%), ADHD (4.7% vs. 1.0%), ASD (4.7% vs. 1.0%), any neurodevelopmental disorder(NDD) (i.e., learning disability, ADHD or ASD) (10.5% vs. 3.1%) and any chronic illness (44.0% vs. 25.0%). Partially vaccinated children had an intermediate position between the fully vaccinated and unvaccinated in regard to several but not all health outcomes. For instance, the partially vaccinated had an intermediate (apparently detrimental) position in terms of allergic rhinitis, ADHD, eczema, and learning disability. In summary, vaccination, nonwhite race, and male gender were significantly associated with NDD after controlling for other factors." Notice the last statement regarding nonwhite male children being most susceptible to neurological disorders. Once again, this echoes the information in the Thompson study that was covered up.(10)

In the second study titled, Health effects in vaccinated versus unvaccinated children, with covariates for breastfeeding status and type of birth, "children from three pediatric medical practices in the United States were used as a convenience sample to compare health outcomes in fully vaccinated (136 children), partially vaccinated (484 children), and completely unvaccinated (945 children) populations. Within the logistic regression models, higher odds ratios were observed within the fully and partially vaccinated groups versus the unvaccinated group for severe allergies, autism, gastrointestinal disorders, asthma, attention deficit disorder (ADD/ADHD), and chronic ear infections.(11)

The third study was a joint project between Vanderbilt University, the University of London and the University of Illinois at Chicago. Information was gathered through the use of a "survey mailed to 2,964 member households of the National Vaccine Information

Center, which represents people concerned about vaccine safety, to ascertain vaccination and atopic disease status. The data included 515 never vaccinated, 423 partially vaccinated, and 239 completely vaccinated children. In multiple regression analyses there were significant and dose-dependent negative relationships between vaccination refusal and self-reported asthma or hay fever only in children with no family history of the condition and, for asthma, in children with no exposure to antibiotics during infancy. Parents who refuse vaccinations reported less asthma and allergies in their unvaccinated children."(12)

Our fourth and final study was recently published in the International *Journal of Vaccine Theory, Practice and Research* by a group calling themselves The Control Group. In 2019-2020 the control group performed a nationwide survey of unvaccinated Americans meant to quantify the long-term health risks of total vaccine avoidance against the health outcomes observed in the 99.74% vaccine-exposed American population. Their findings? "The null hypothesis, that no significant difference would be found between vaccinated vs. unvaccinated persons in heart disease, diabetes, digestive disorders, eczema, asthma, allergies, developmental disabilities, birth defects, epilepsy, autism, ADHD, cancers, and arthritis, is rejected with overwhelming statistical confidence and power in every single contrast." The author concluded the paper by stating, "Vaccines are NOT moving the population toward better health, as suggested by the World Health Organization and the US Department of Health & Human Services, but rather toward epidemic levels of lifelong debilitating chronic disorders." (13) Regarding this survey, statistician Jan-Willem van der Bergh stated, "The differences in health outcomes between the population of entirely unvaccinated and vaccine exposed are staggering." He went on to state that, "There is very strong evidence, with a probability near 100%...that these illness rates are accurate."

When you look at all of the studies I have placed here they tell a singular story; vaccines are not the panacea that they are being presented as and anything that has the potential consequences that these drugs have should not be mandated to our children. The vaccine apologists will undoubtedly tear these studies to pieces with an untold number of criticisms. Some of the criticisms could be valid just as many of the criticisms that go against studies that purport to validate vaccines as safe and effective are as well. Bottom line is there needs to be more studies done that involve large numbers of children. These studies need to be done on two groups: one receiving all of the vaccines currently mandated and the other receiving none of these vaccines. These groups then need to be followed and monitored closely for an extended period of time (say 10 years). These studies would most likely be the only way to finally put to bed all of the questions that exist regarding the safety concerns and long-term effects of vaccines. Lastly, this study would need to either be done by some completely independent research body or by a panel that includes an equal number of scientists from both sides of this contentious issue. This would ensure that both parties come away from the study satisfied with the results and leaving no one to criticize the outcome. However, as I stated at the beginning of this Point, they have to want to see the results to agree to a study such as this. I hate to sound completely pessimistic but I highly doubt that this day will ever come. The consequences for the vaccine apologists are far too risky for them to ever agree to a study that even remotely looks like the one I described. So they will continue to deny the issues; attempt to destroy the reputations of any scientist who participates in any research that says the wrong things; and bad mouth any research that contradicts their script. This is their game and they will stick to it no matter what happens. Your job then, if you choose to accept it, is to do the deep dive yourself and put the pieces together.

Point Number Ten
Vaccine Schedules

"Differences challenge assumptions."
~ Anne Wilson Schaef, American clinical psychologist and author

If I had a dime for every time someone said, "Hey, I had my vaccines when I was a kid and nothing happened to me," I would be a very wealthy man. Two very big problems exist with that statement. The first problem would be that just because something does not happen to one individual does not mean it can not happen to another individual. Will everyone have an adverse reaction to a drug? The answer to that is a definitive no. Yet adverse events to drugs occur regularly. The second problem with that original statement is that depending on the age of the person making that statement, their experience with the vaccine schedule could be, and often is, a completely different experience.

Most people who have made that comment to me were born sometime between 1960 and 1980. For those individuals we are not just talking about a comparison of apples and oranges, but more like apples and automobiles. The vaccine schedule then compared to what it is now is not even comparable. Prior to around 1985, you would have only received three vaccines. Those vaccines being the DTP, MMR and Polio vaccines. Of course two of those vaccines are combinations (Diphtheria-Tetanus-Pertussis and the Measles-Mumps-Rubella) so the total number of diseases you were immunized against was seven.(1) By the time 1985 rolled around the amount had only increased by one more vaccine, Hepatitis B (Hib).(2) Then something occurred which radically changed the entire makeup of the vaccination program. In 1986 the National Childhood Injury Act (NCIA) (through intense encouragement by pharmaceutical companies) was enacted by Congress and through this the National Vaccine Injury Compensation Program (NVICP) was developed. The radical change created was that the NVICP "provides that no vaccine manufacturer shall be liable in a civil action for damages arising from a vaccine-related injury or death: 1. resulting from unavoidable side effects; or 2. solely due to the manufacturer's failure to provide direct warnings."(3) Is it any wonder that with no liability against them the vaccine manufacturers began introducing more vaccines for mandatory use for our children than ever before in history? As of 2022, the CDC's childhood vaccine schedule includes more than 30 injections of 14 different vaccines.(4) As if this were not enough, there are currently, a total of 2,612 vaccines being investigated for a number of infectious diseases. (5) Can you fathom what the mandatory list of vaccinations might look like in another decade?

You will hear the vaccine apologists say that all of the vaccines in the schedule have gone through rigorous research to show that they are safe and effective. While each of the individual vaccines have undergone research to prove their safety (see Point 7 to understand the validity of the science) there is one vaccine study that has never been done. This one vaccine, that has never been studied and needs to be in order to show what actually happens when a child gets their full complement of vaccines, is the "DiphtheriaTetanusPertussisMeaslesMumpsRubellaPolioHibHepatitisBVaricellaHepatitisAPneumococcalInfluenzaRotavirus" vaccine. In other words, there has never been any comprehensive study to look at the effects of the entire vaccine schedule on an individual. When a child is getting more than 30 injections of 14 different vaccines there is a very complex situation occurring inside of this child. It is likely not a singular vaccine that is causing the issues that so many are concerned with. It is far more likely that the cascade of events unfolding within a child's body when they are injected with so many vaccines is where the real answer will be found. During the same time period that the vaccine schedule has been increasing exponentially, we also have autoimmune diseases, autism, type 1 diabetes mellitus, allergies, infant mortality and more also rising exponentially.(6,7,8,9,10) Coincidence, could be, or perhaps there is an environmental cause that affects all children that could be creating these problems. What environmental link would affect nearly 90% of all children in the U.S.? Could it be vaccines? Until we do the proper studies we will never know.

"Studies designed to examine the long-term effects of the cumulative number of vaccines or other aspects of the immunization schedule have not been conducted." This quote comes directly from the Institutes of Medicine in a book released in 2013 by the National Academies Press and titled The Childhood Immunization Schedule and Safety (Summary, pg 6). Unfortunately, as is all too familiar, we do not have the studies we need to be able to connect the dots to these issues and concerns, so we must look at the studies we have. The following studies all show the effects on children from the vaccine schedule as it is given. These studies illustrate the potential connections to multiple injections of vaccines and a long list of adverse events.

One of the best blood markers we have that measures the general amount of inflammation in your body is C-reactive protein (CRP). In this first study, the researchers used blood levels of CRP to look at the effects of multiple vaccines on children. "Abnormal elevation of CRP level occurred in 85% of infants administered multiple vaccines and up to 70% of those given a single vaccine. Overall, 16% of infants had vaccine-associated cardiorespiratory events within 48 hours post immunization. In logistic regression analysis, abnormal CRP values were associated with multiple vaccines and severe intraventricular hemorrhage (IVH). Cardiorespiratory events were associated marginally with receipt of multiple injections and significantly with gastroesophageal reflux (GER). Underlying medical conditions and possibly multiple injections are associated with cardiorespiratory events."(11)

This second study included over 56,000 children. Their goal was to see if the cumulative effects of adjuvants from multiple vaccines was linked with type 2 immunity which is commonly seen in allergic responses. "We hypothesized that cumulative adjuvant exposure in infancy may influence the development of allergies later in life by changing the balance of type 1/type 2 immunity. Physician-diagnosed asthma was associated with receiving three or four to five different inactivated vaccines, compared with children who received only one inactivated vaccine. Similar results were found for two questionnaire-based symptoms, i.e. wheeze (three vaccines vs. a single vaccine) and eczema (four or five vaccines vs. a single vaccine). Our results, which should be cautiously interpreted, suggest that the prevalence of asthma, wheeze and eczema among children at 12 months of age might be related to the amount of inactivated vaccine exposure before 6 months of age."(12)

In this third study the researchers looked at the usage of three vaccines in a group of over 4,000 children in a rural area of Senegal. "At 12 months the vaccination coverage was 44%, 46% and 9%, respectively, for BCG, DTP1 and MV. Most children received BCG+DTP1-first and this combination was associated with a significantly lower mortality rate ratio (MRR) of 0.69 compared with unvaccinated children. There was no benefit for children receiving BCG-first or DTP1-first. The female-male MRR was 0.79 among unvaccinated children, but was significantly inversed with 1.45 for children receiving DTP vaccination. Children who had received DTP simultaneously with MV or DTP after MV had significantly higher mortality (MRR=2.59) compared with children having MV-only as their most recent vaccination. After 9 months, the female-male MRR was 0.61 for measles-vaccinated children but remained 1.54 for DTP-vaccinated children who had not received MV. The sequence of routine vaccinations is important for the overall impact on child survival and these vaccines are associated with sex-differential effects."(13) Notice how significantly the mortality increased along with the number of vaccines given.

The group of researchers in this study performed a longitudinal, case-control pilot study "that examined amygdala growth in rhesus macaque infants receiving the complete US childhood vaccine schedule (1994-1999). Vaccine-exposed and saline-injected control infants underwent MRI and PET imaging at approximately four and six months of age, representing two specific timeframes within the vaccine schedule. These results suggest that maturational changes in amygdala volume and the binding capacity of diprenorphine (DPN) in the amygdala was significantly altered in infant macaques receiving the vaccine schedule." (14) The findings of this study allude to a role that the vaccine schedule may have in affecting the amygdala which plays a major role in emotional regulation. The inability for proper emotional regulation is a hallmark feature in autism.

In this next study the authors wanted to look directly at the increase in infant mortality and what possible role the vaccine schedule may play. The US childhood immunization schedule (from 2011) requires 26 vaccine doses for infants aged less than one year, the most in the world, yet 33 nations have better Infant Mortality Rates (IMRs). Using linear regression, the immunization schedules of these 34 nations were examined and a correlation coefficient of 0.70 was found between IMRs and the number of vaccine doses routinely given to infants. When nations were grouped into five different vaccine dose ranges (12–14, 15–17, 18–20, 21–23, and 24–26), 98.3% of the total variance in IMR was explained by the unweighted linear regression model. These findings demonstrate a counter-intuitive relationship: nations that require more vaccine doses tend to have higher infant mortality rates.(15)

When we talk about science, one of the items discussed will inevitably be animal studies. Here are two animal studies showing the adverse effects of multiple vaccines. The first one was performed on 1,226,159 dogs vaccinated at 360 veterinary hospitals and the second study was done on 496,189 cats vaccinated at 329 hospitals. "The risk of a vaccine-associated adverse event (VAAE) significantly increased as the number of vaccine doses administered per office visit increased; each additional vaccine significantly increased risk of an adverse event by 27% in dogs ≤ 10 kg (22 lb) and 12% in dogs > 10 kg. Young adult small-breed neutered dogs that received multiple vaccines per office visit were at greatest risk of a VAAE within 72 hours after vaccination."(16) "The risk of a vaccine-associated adverse events (VAAE) significantly increased as the number of vaccines administered per office visit increased. Risk was greatest for cats approximately 1year old.

Veterinarians should incorporate these findings into risk communications and limit the number of vaccinations administered concurrently to cats."(17)

The researchers in this next study looked at a total of 38,787 adverse events reported to the Vaccine Adverse Events Reporting System (VAERS) during the period 1991-1994. VAERS is a self-reporting, passive surveillance system. We already know that approximately 1% of all events get reported so any numbers we see in research like this is likely far higher than the research reports. "Adverse events with onset of symptoms the day of vaccination accounted for 45.5% of total reports; 20.4% had onset of symptoms the following day. Onset within 2 weeks after vaccination was noted for 92.5% of all reports. Simultaneous administration of multiple vaccines was noted in 75.7% of reports for immunizations at ages younger than 20 years. In contrast, among those 20 years or older, only 6.0% of reports named multiple vaccines."(18)

In a similar study looking at the Vaccine Adverse Event Reporting System (VAERS) database, this time from the period 1990-2010, the authors looked for a correlation between the number of vaccines given and hospitalizations and death. "Cases that specified either hospitalization or death were identified among 38,801 reports of infants. The hospitalization rate increased linearly from 11.0% for 2 doses to 23.5% for 8 doses. The rate ratio (RR) of the mortality rate for 5-8 vaccine doses to 1-4 vaccine doses is 1.5, indicating a statistically significant increase from 3.6% deaths associated with 1-4 vaccine doses to 5.5% associated with 5-8 vaccine doses. Our findings show a positive correlation between the number of vaccine doses administered and the percentage of hospitalizations and deaths.(19) Different studies with almost identical outcomes.

The final study we will look at came from researchers from the Kaiser Permanente Institute for Health Research. Their goal: "To examine patterns and trends of undervaccination in children aged 2 to 24 months and to compare health care utilization rates between undervaccinated and age-appropriately vaccinated children." They took their information from "children born between 2004 and 2008" gathered from "eight managed care organizations of the Vaccine Safety Datalink." "Children who were undervaccinated because of parental choice had lower rates of outpatient visits and emergency department encounters than age-appropriately vaccinated children."(20) The children in this study ranged greatly in the number of vaccines received. Those that received less than the recommended vaccine schedule were considered "undervaccinated." So these were not truly unvaccinated children being compared to vaccinated ones but instead they were children who received the full schedule versus those that did not receive the full schedule. Once again we end up with an outcome that places those who have received a greater number of vaccines in a worse outcome over those who received less vaccines.

Although all of these studies grouped together still do not supply absolute verifiable proof that the vaccine schedule is to blame for the issues mentioned in them, it certainly creates questions that need answers. It also makes crystal clear that the continued statements that the vaccine apologists make regarding how safe the vaccines are and how "all" of the research proves this idea, is a completely false statement. There have been a few unvaccinated versus vaccinated studies that, though the studies are not large enough nor detailed enough to illustrate everything we need, still have shown the same outcomes as we have seen here in our discussion. The unvaccinated children have less allergies, less neurodevelopmental issues, less chronic illness, etc. (21,22,23) I believe that most parents do not realize that they have the freedom (currently) to refuse vaccines altogether. Also if they do not have the inclination to refuse all vaccines outright there are also alternative schedules that they could choose.(24) These alternative schedules would allow you to either space out all of the scheduled vaccines across a longer time table or skip certain vaccines while choosing others. Unfortunately, it is doubtful that you will find many pediatricians letting their patients know any of that.

Understanding the potential risks that come with vaccination is one of the most important things a parent (or for that matter any individual) needs to know. The increase of the vaccine schedule and the concurrent increase in so many childhood problems should be concerning to everyone. Although the vaccine apologists will repeat the story that a child's immune system can handle all of the vaccines in the current schedule and more. In fact, they will tell you that a child's immune system is strengthened by vaccines.(25) It should not take much thinking before understanding how ridiculous those statements sound. A newborn infant's immune system is as immature as the child itself and takes a while to fully develop.(26) The absurd notion that injecting a child's developing immune system, nervous system and every other system with 30 injections of 14 different diseases and expecting nothing adverse to occur is the script upon which all of the vaccine apologists ideals are placed. And it is this story that they are depending on parents buying into.

Point Number Eleven
Dr Andrew Wakefield

"When we believe in lies, we cannot see the truth, so we make thousands of assumptions and we take them as truth. One of the biggest assumptions we make is that the lies we believe are the truth!"
~Don Miguel Ruiz, Author

I would like to begin this Point by stating that Dr. Wakefield does not need my defense of him. In fact, I do not really know Dr. Wakefield personally. We have met only once before at a seminar and I found him to be a very intelligent and compassionate man. The reason for having a Point specifically for him is because of how often he is brought up as something any good "antivaxxer" should be ashamed of. He is also an excellent example of what the pharmaceutical companies and the media shills do to anyone who questions vaccines. I am not sure exactly why the vaccine apologists ever thought that continually bad mouthing the good doctor would have some kind of positive outcome, but yet they still do. Just type his name into your search engine and see what comes up. Google will give you page after page of very negative information all of it centering on two things: "disgraced doctor who had study retracted" and "antivaxx leader." Is he either of these two things? Let's look at the first label they have tried to pin on Dr. Wakefield.

If you bring up Dr. Wakefield it is amazing how many people will have this immediate visceral, negative reaction. It is equally amazing how many of these same individuals know nothing about this man or the story around this paper except for what the media wants them to know. Yet they will go down in flames defending this information as if they themselves did a deep dive into the information and know it all to be factual. Well, I can tell you that I have done the deep dive into this subject and can tell you that it is incredibly easy to sit in judgment of another and assume their quilt. It is quite another thing altogether to take the time it requires to investigate the information you are being fed to ensure that the individual in question is being represented fairly. All of the character attacks of Dr. Wakefield began back in 1998 when he and 12 other doctors wrote and published a paper titled Ileal-lymphoid-nodular hyperplasia, non-specific colitis, and pervasive developmental disorder in children. Because this paper revealed a possible link between the MMR vaccine and autism it immediately became a flashpoint for this issue. The paper was eventually retracted by the *BMJ* in Feb. of 2010 and six months later Dr. Wakefield's license to practice medicine in Britain was revoked.

The General Medical Council (GMC) (of the UK) made the decision to revoke Dr. Wakefield's license based on multiple grounds. I went into my investigation into this information with an open mind. I was willing to accept his full guilt if that was what the information revealed to me. What I found was a collection of mis-truths, half-truths and speculation. What I didn't find was anything that would make me feel the actions against Dr. Wakefield were warranted. This does not mean that I am a legal expert nor for that matter a research expert. I am however someone who can look at information critically and decipher said information to come to a reasonable conclusion. Look at the information and make your judgments on this individual based, not on what one media source tells you, but information from all sources. Let's look at a few of the claims raised against Dr. Wakefield.

1. The study claimed that there was a link between the administration of the measles, mumps and rubella (MMR) vaccine, and the appearance of autism and bowel disease. This statement is found on almost every single search result that you will bring up. Every news report or vaccine apologists website seems to use this exact same statement. However, all you need do is go to the actual paper and see that this is not at all what the paper claimed. "We investigated a consecutive series of children with chronic enterocolitis and regressive developmental disorder." "No association was made with

the vaccine at this time." "We did not prove an association between measles, mumps, and rubella vaccine and the syndrome described. Virological studies are underway that may help to resolve this issue." "Published evidence is inadequate to show whether there is a change in incidence or a link with measles, mumps, and rubella vaccine." "In most cases, onset of symptoms was after measles, mumps, and rubella immunization."(1) Clearly the paper does not make the claim that the vast majority of search results state it does. Even in a video press release from the Royal Free hospital where Dr. Wakefield and some of his fellow researchers were brought to answer questions regarding the paper; his answers were very clear about not placing blame or trying to incite panic. Read the following excerpts from the interview (ironically taken from the website of Dr. Wakefield's biggest critic):

INTERVIEWER: There has been concern recently over any long term effects as a result of the MMR vaccine, are you saying now then that there does appear to be a proven link between the vaccine and the side effects?

DR ANDREW WAKEFIELD: No, the work certainly raises a question mark over MMR vaccine, but as it is, there is no proven link as such and we are seeking to establish whether there is a genuine causal association between the MMR and this syndrome or not. It is our suspicion that there may well be but that is far from being a causal association that is proven beyond doubt.

INTERVIEWER: But if you say there's at least a question mark over it now, should the vaccine continue to be administered while you're investigating?

DR ANDREW WAKEFIELD: I think if you asked members of the team that have investigated this they would give you different answers. And I have to say that there is sufficient anxiety in my own mind of the safety, the long term safety of the polyvalent, that is the MMR vaccination in combination, that I think that it should be suspended in favor of the single vaccines, that is continued use of the individual measles, mumps and rubella components.(2)

He continues in this fashion through the rest of his part of the interview. Each time he is asked a pointed question regarding the vaccine and autism he carefully and thoughtfully declines to state a clear connection and when asked further regarding the usage of the vaccine he again calmly and clearly states that he is only giving his opinion and that he is not saying to not get vaccinated. There can be no question based on the actual paper nor in his interview prior to the publication of the paper that his intent was ever to stop people from getting vaccinations or that he and his colleagues had found a causal link to autism.

2. Dr. Wakefield had two major conflicts of interest; one was that he had a patent on a potential rival MMR vaccine and the other was that he was being paid by lawyers to represent vaccine injured children. Here again are two bits of information that will be found in essentially every negative article written about him and again the facts are not as dastardly as they attempt to make them out to be. Let's address the first accusation; his patent. Dr. wakefield along with Dr. H. Hugh Fudenberg, an immunologist and former professor and chairman of the department of basic and clinical immunology and microbiology with the Medical University of South Carolina, are listed on this patent as inventors while it is the Royal Free Hospital that is listed as the applicant and therefore the actual holder of the patent.(3) If the idea of being a part of a medical patent was truly evil and offensive to the vaccine apologists, then you would think that they would be equally offended at the CDC being one of the largest patent owners in this arena. (4)(5) In fact, Dr. Paul Offit, widely seen as one of the most vocal vaccine apologists on record, is a patent owner himself. When asked by a UPI reporter about conflicts of interest in the vaccine process his response was, "I am probably just the kind of person you are talking about," said Paul Offit, chief of infectious diseases at the Children's Hospital of Philadelphia, who was a committee member until last month. At the same time, he shared a patent for another rotavirus vaccine. Merck has funded Offit's research for 13 years. "I am a co-holder of a patent for a (rotavirus) vaccine. If this vaccine were to become a routinely recommended vaccine, I would make money off of that," Offit said. "When I review safety data,

am I biased? That answer is really easy: absolutely not." "Is there an unholy alliance between the people who make recommendations about vaccines and the vaccine manufacturers? The answer is no." Merck bought and delivered copies of Offit's book, *What Every Parent Should Know About Vaccines*, to American doctors. The book has a list price of $14.95. "Merck Vaccine Division is pleased to present you with a copy of the recent publication, 'What Every Parent Should Know About Vaccines,'" says a Dear Doctor letter from Merck. "The authors designed the book to answer questions parents have about vaccines and to dispel misinformation about vaccines that sometimes appears in the public media. Offit said he does not know how many copies of his book Merck purchased. "I don't have any control over that," he said."(6) So one of the biggest spokesperson for the pharmaceutical industry owns a vaccine patent (by the way he holds six patents) is funded by big pharma for research that he performs and is getting paid from pharmaceutical companies selling his book for him. So while I do not agree with any scientist having a financial situation that could potentially sway their judgment, you can not hold a double standard and say that one person should be condemned for it while another is acceptable. Which is exactly what the vaccine apologists are doing. On the matter of being paid by the lawyers, all of the evidence I have seen shows that the timing of the paper and the payments do not show a clear line of deceit. Dr. Wakefield's own testimony clearly states that the money he received came after the paper was completed and was not involved in the paper in question.(7) The 55,000 pounds that Dr. Wakefield was "paid" by the lawyer went directly towards a separate study that started after the *Lancet* paper and he did not personally benefit from this payment. The practice of medical doctors being paid to be expert witnesses is a common one and is not illegal or immoral. In a letter written to The Highwire, the lawyer in question, Richard Barr, stated that the study "was not funded by Legal Aid and (was) not part of the litigation."(8) Even one of the studies co-authors went on record saying, "I don't think there was any conflict of interest" and that he (the author) still would have put his name on the study.(9) What should be the final point on this subject is that the editors of the *Lancet* knew of Dr. Wakefield's role with the lawsuit and were ok with his position prior to publishing the paper.(10)

3. Ethics approval was never given to perform invasive testing on the children in the study. All approval that was needed was acquired and approved by the Royal Free Hospital as stated in the approved final paper. As this paper was primarily a series of case reports, ethical approval was not necessary beyond what Prof. Walker-Smith, who was the senior co-author on the paper, had already received. In a statement by the editors of the *Lancet* that was published upon receiving the allegations against the authors of this paper they stated, "The evidence we have seen indicates that ethics committee approval was given for data collection from clinically indicated investigations in the children with an initially undiagnosed illness and who were described in the 1998 *Lancet* paper."(10)

4. Dr. Wakefield hand selected the children involved in the study therefore biasing the outcome. I will once again defer to the editors of the *Lancet* in their response to the allegations: "Professor Walker-Smith notes that although the referral pattern was unusual—direct contact by patients with Dr Wakefield leading to referral to the Royal Free—the children were indeed consecutively referred. He reports that to the best of his recollection he did not invite any children to participate in the study. Thus, as far as the facts can be ascertained by a review of the case notes and from memory, children reported in the 1998 *Lancet* paper were consecutively referred to the Royal Free and were not deliberately sought by the authors for inclusion in their study based on parents' beliefs about an association between their child's illness and the MMR vaccine."(10) Dr. Wakefield himself goes into detail involving the selection process of the children for this study in his affidavit.(7)

5. Dr. Wakefield's actions led to increased outbreaks and deaths from measles in the UK. Another piece of the script that multiple media sources have used in their denigration of Dr. Wakefield.(11)(12)(13)(14) This one is so incredibly easy to disprove that it clearly illustrates the lack of investigation into what is the truth in this

story. One look at the UK government's own website records of measles infections and deaths tells the story is completely false.(15) Infection rates in 1998 were 3,728 with 3 deaths reported. Those infection rates never went above the 1998 numbers until 2008 and death rates never exceeded the 3 in 1998 until 2019. Any claims that this paper created some dire consequence is hyperbole at best and outright lies at worst.

Another item that the vaccine apologists love to state as a fact is that Dr. Wakefield's research (by the way there were 12 others involved in the retracted paper) has never been reproduced and has been proven to be false. Understand that Dr. Wakefield had begun looking into the possible connection between measles, MMR and gut issues such as irritable bowel and Crohn's disease before the infamous retracted study was published in 1998. Here are some studies that had already been published prior to the Wakefield paper and more since:

- 1991 "Granulomatous Vasculitis in Crohn's Disease." "The results suggest that the majority of granulomas in Crohn's disease form within walls of blood vessels. Vascular localization of granulomatous inflammation suggests that the intestinal microvasculature contains an early element in the pathogenesis of Crohn's disease." Though not related to measles, this is to illustrate his focus on this subject material well before '98.(16)

- 1993 "Evidence of persistent measles virus infection in Crohn's disease." "These observations suggest that measles virus is capable of causing persistent infection of the intestine and that Crohn's disease may be caused by a granulomatous vasculitis in response to this virus."(17)

- 1995 "Is Measles Vaccination a Risk Factor for Inflammatory Bowel Disease?" "Prevalences of Crohn's disease, ulcerative colitis, coeliac disease, and peptic ulceration were determined in 3545 people who had received live measles vaccine in 1964 as part of a measles vaccine trial. A longitudinal birth cohort of 11407 subjects was one unvaccinated comparison cohort, and 2541 partners of those vaccinated was another. These findings suggest that measles virus may play a part in the development not only of Crohn's disease but also of ulcerative colitis."(18)

- 1995 "Detection of immunoreactive antigen, with a monoclonal antibody to measles virus, in tissue from a patient with Crohn's disease." "The role of measles virus infection and/or a viral antigen (possibly the M protein) as a causative agent in Crohn's disease poses a challenging avenue for further research."(19)

- 2000 "Enterocolitis in children with developmental disorders." "Chronic colitis was identified in 53 of 60 (88%) affected children compared with one of 22 (4.5%) controls and in 20 of 20 (100%) with Ulcerative Colitis. A new variant of inflammatory bowel disease is present in this group of children with developmental disorders."(20)

- 2000 "Detection and Sequencing of Measles Virus from Peripheral Mononuclear Cells from Patients with Inflammatory Bowel Disease and Autism." "The sequences obtained from the patients with Crohn's disease shared the characteristics with wild-strain virus. The sequences obtained from the patients with ulcerative colitis and children with autism were consistent with being vaccine strains. The results were concordant with the exposure history of the patients. Persistence of measles virus was confirmed in PBMC in some patients with chronic intestinal inflammation."(21)

- 2001 "Colonic CD8 and γδ T-cell infiltration with epithelial damage in children with autism." "Immunohistochemistry confirms a distinct lymphocytic colitis in autistic spectrum disorders in which the epithelium appears particularly affected. This is consistent with increasing evidence for gut epithelial dysfunction in autism."(22)

- 2001 "Measles is more prevalent in Crohn's disease patients. A multicentre Israeli study." "These data lead us to postulate that that there may be a role for measles infection in Crohn's disease, even if, at present, this role remains unclear."(23)

- 2002 "The concept of entero-colonic encephalopathy, autism and opioid receptor ligands." "The various concepts explored in this review are capable of generating an abundance of hypotheses, most of which are testable in clinical and laboratory settings. Initially, however, a comprehensive quantitative and qualitative characterization of opioid (endogenous and exogenous) profiles is merited, in the blood, urine and cerebrospinal fluid of phenotypically homogeneous groups of children with autism, both on and off exclusion diets, including matched controls."(24)

- 2002 "Potential viral pathogenic mechanism for new variant inflammatory bowel disease." "Seventy five of 91 patients with a histologically confirmed diagnosis of ileal lymphonodular hyperplasia and enterocolitis were positive for measles virus in their intestinal tissue compared with five of 70 control patients. The data confirm an association between the presence of measles virus and gut pathology in children with developmental disorder."(25)

- 2003 "Intestinal Lymphocyte Populations in Children with Regressive Autism: Evidence for Extensive Mucosal Immunopathology." "The data provide further evidence of a pan-enteric mucosal immunopathology in children with regressive autism that is apparently distinct from other inflammatory bowel diseases."(26)

- 2004 "Spontaneous Mucosal Lymphocyte Cytokine Profiles in Children with Autism and Gastrointestinal Symptoms: Mucosal Immune Activation and Reduced Counter Regulatory Interleukin-10." "The data provide further evidence of a diffuse mucosal immunopathology in some ASD children and the potential for benefit of dietary and immunomodulatory therapies."(27)

- 2006 "Immune activation of peripheral blood and mucosal CD3+ lymphocyte cytokine profiles in children with autism and gastrointestinal symptoms." "There is a unique pattern of peripheral blood and mucosal CD3+ lymphocytes intracellular cytokines, which is consistent with significant immune dysregulation, in this ASD cohort."(28)

- 2016 "Infectious, atopic and inflammatory diseases, childhood adversities and familial aggregation are independently associated with the risk for mental disorders: Results from a large Swiss epidemiological study." "Associations with infectious, atopic and other chronic inflammatory diseases were observable together with consistent effects of childhood adversities and familial aggregation, and less consistent effects of trauma in each group of mental disorders. Gastric inflammatory diseases took effect in mood disorders (both sexes) and in early disorders (men). Similarly, irritable bowel syndrome was prominent..."(29)

- 2019 "Role of the Gut Microbiome in Autism Spectrum Disorders." "A gut disorder akin to Crohn's disease is, sometimes, reported in autistic children, an extremely painful gastrointestinal disease which is named as autistic enterocolitis. This disturbed situation hypothesized to be initiated by dysbiosis or microbial imbalance could in turn perturb the coordination of microbiota-gut-brain axis which is important in human mental health as goes the popular dictum: "fix your gut, fix your brain."(30)

- 2020 "Environmental exposures and the risk of inflammatory bowel disease: a case-control study from Saudi Arabia." "receiving seven vaccines or more during childhood increased the risk of developing inflammatory bowel disease by nine-fold."(31)

Clearly the statements that the original ideas in the 1998 *Lancet* paper were never reproduced and that the concepts contained within them were proven false is not quite what it seems. James Lyons-Weiler, PHD, the author of a fantastic book titled *The Environmental and Genetic Causes of Autism,* mentions that one of the limitations of the original 1998 *Lancet* study was the sole focus on the MMR vaccine without even considering that there could be influences from other vaccines as well. He covers several plausible gut connections with autism in his book with research that supports his conclusions. The other idea that articles continuously tie to the paper and Dr. Wakefield is the whole MMR-Autism connection. First, I have already shown that was not the objective of the paper and as for "no connection to autism," simply go back to Point 8 to see how accurate that piece of the script actually is.

As mentioned earlier, there were 13 scientists that were a part of the 1998 *Lancet* paper. The news reports will tell you that ten of the thirteen retracted their support for the study. So what did they say exactly, "The main thrust of this paper was the first description of an unexpected intestinal lesion in the children reported. Further evidence has been forthcoming in studies from the Royal Free Centre for Paediatric Gastroenterology and other groups to support and extend these findings. While much uncertainty remains about the nature of these changes, we believe it important that such work continues, as autistic children can potentially be helped by recognition and treatment of gastrointestinal problems. We wish to make it clear that in this paper no causal link was established between MMR vaccine and autism as the data were insufficient. However, the possibility of such a link was raised and consequent events have had major implications for public health. In view of this, we consider now is the appropriate time that we should together formally retract the interpretation placed upon these findings in the paper, according to precedent."(32) While it is true that the co-authors of the paper withdrew their support for the study's interpretations, it is not, however, true to conclude that, as the news articles state, they retracted their support of the study. The co-authors make a clear distinct point that they stand by the paper's content, but not the interpretations made after publication. Realize that all of the authors had to sign off on the study before it was published. Only two of the thirteen doctors connected to this paper were punished by loss of license, Dr. Wakefield and Prof. Walker-Smith. Prof. Walker-Smith went forward with an appeal of the decision. While Prof. Walker-Smith was funded in his appeal, Dr. Wakefield was not, making it financially impossible for him to appeal the decision. Prof. Walker-Smith eventually won his appeal. "Mr Justice Mitting, sitting at the high court in London, ruled that the GMC decision "cannot stand". He quashed the 2010 finding of professional misconduct and the striking off. Calling for changes in the way GMC fitness to practice panel hearings are conducted , the judge said of the flawed handling of Walker-Smith's case: "It would be a misfortune if this were to happen again."(33)

Further complicating the charges, the editor of the *Lancet*, Richard Horton, "still considers the paper important because it identified a new syndrome suffered by children who had symptoms both of chronic bowel disease and autism. "I do not regret for one second publishing details of this new syndrome," he said. "I'm disappointed that Liam Donaldson [chief medical officer] has stated this was poor science. By stating that, he dismisses a very important novel observation."(34) Further confounding the decision to penalize Dr. Wakefield as they did, "David Lewis [a microbiologist and] of the National Whistleblower's Center in Washington DC published a letter in the *BMJ* (http://bmj.com) arguing that Wakefield did not commit research fraud. Lewis told *Nature* that he thinks the combination of public charges and a slow, secretive investigation has left the public not knowing whom to believe and is unfair to the accused researcher. "[The system] throws people like Andy into a no-man's-land," Lewis says."(35) Mr. Lewis came to his conclusions after reviewing files given to him by Dr. Wakefield. "The *BMJ* asked Ingvar Bjarnason, a gastroenterologist at King's College Hospital, London, to review the materials. He says that the forms don't clearly support charges that Wakefield deliberately misinterpreted the records. "The data are subjective. It's different to say it's deliberate falsification," he says."(35)

Dr. Andrew Wakefield is but one example of a doctor persecuted for speaking out against the vaccine ideology. There are a multitude of doctors and scientists who have been attacked, vilified, demonized and destroyed because their opinions or ideas did not conform to the script.(36)(37)(38)(39)(40)(41)(42)(43)(44) Others are speaking out over the issue of doctors being attacked, "Justice Centre Litigation Director Jay Cameron also has concern over the growing censorship of medical professionals when it comes to questioning the government narrative on Covid. "We are seeing a clear pattern of highly competent and skilled medical doctors in very esteemed positions being taken down and censored or even fired, for practicing proper science and medicine," says Mr. Cameron."(44) "Given reports that doctors and other medical professionals are being silenced about coronavirus conditions, the country's two largest physician groups say doctors have the right to be heard. Both the American Medical Association (AMA) and the American College of Physicians (ACP) issued statements

Wednesday supporting the rights of physicians to speak out on COVID-19 care conditions."(45)

As to the idea that somehow Dr. Wakefield is the leader of the "anti-vax" movement, this is easily shown as hyperbole. People standing against the idea of mandatory vaccines has been occurring since mandatory vaccines began. Protests are on record as occurring as early as the 1800s. (46) Individuals in the forefront of this movement have been many over this time period, with no singular person really standing out as a leader. In the 1970's, Dr. Gordon Stewart, published a series of case reports linking neurological disorders to DTP and became a focal point for concerned parents everywhere. Barbara Loe-Fisher was someone who came to the fore in the 90's when her book *A Shot in the Dark* was published. She quickly became one of the most vocal people for vaccine changes in Washington DC. Other people have stood out over the years as singular voices, however the vast majority of what has occurred in this movement has been led by parents, mainly the mothers of vaccine injured children. If there is a "leader" in the movement for medical freedom it is the thousands of mothers who have been fighting the good fight for their children all of these years.

So what's the conclusion here? Is Dr. Wakefield a fraud? Is he the head of the anti-vaxx movement? I can only tell you what I know from all of my research, Dr. Andrew Wakefield is a very intelligent, dedicated doctor and researcher. He cares deeply about the issues with children that he has spent a large part of his life researching. The case against him is a straw house. Evidence from affidavit and testimony from a variety of sources all refute the versions that the GMC seemed to utilize in making their decisions. It is necessary to understand that the GMC is not a "judge and jury" situation but instead is a body of lay people and professionals who hear information and then make a decision. Not necessarily a legal decision but their opinion is final. Why did they decide the way they did? I could string together theories of conspiracy and questionable motives, but that still does nothing to really answer why all of this has played out the way that it has. The idea that there is some large income waiting for someone who questions vaccine ideas is certainly a false one. By going against the vaccine script you immediately set yourself up for persecution by the medical establishment. The media, which gets an enormous portion of its funding through pharma and the medical model then begins slamming you with puff pieces approved by their sponsors. To say that someone chooses to go this route because they think they are going to get rich or acquire fame is not thinking the idea through very well. Dr. Wakefield would have far more money and far more opportunities to become well known in his field if he had simply not rocked the boat. Thankfully he chose to be true to his conscience and his morals. My hope is that more people will do their own deeper look into this story so that he may one day be looked at with the respect he deserves instead of buying into the narrative they are being presented with.

Point Number Twelve
Herd Immunity

"The dissenter is every human being at those moments of his life when he resigns momentarily from the herd and thinks for himself."
~Archibald MacLeish, American poet and writer

If ever an individual suggests the outrageous idea that they should have the right to choose whether or not they or their children should get vaccinated, the almost immediate outcry is "herd immunity!" The idea of the individual protecting the "herd" through the sacrificing of their individual rights seems to be a central point for the moral high ground of the pro-vaxxer. It is the speaking point by which just about every person who is in favor of vaccines will eventually come back to every time. We must protect the herd! It seems like a nice sentiment, but is it accurate? Does this concept of herd immunity really operate the way that most people think it does? It is yet again, another example of a talking point that most people have not investigated thoroughly prior to staking their entire argument on it. Let's break it down, shall we.

The term "herd immunity" has been utilized for a long time now. "The earliest use of the phrase [herd immunity] can be traced to a 1917 report from the US Bureau of Animal Industry that dealt with a cattle infection causing death of unborn calves. A cow that had aborted was likely to become immune, and calves born and raised in such an affected herd were tolerant to the disease."(1) Even though we have been utilizing this term for such a long time, it seems to have some confusion as to its exact usage or meaning among scientists and authors. "Some authors use it to describe the proportion of immune among individuals in a population. Others use it with reference to a particular threshold proportion of immune individuals that should lead to a decline in incidence of infection. Still others use it to refer to a pattern of immunity that should protect a population from invasion of a new infection. A common implication of the term is that the risk of infection among susceptible individuals in a population is reduced by the presence and proximity of immune individuals (this is sometimes referred to as "indirect protection" or a "herd effect")."(2) One of the research papers most often cited by other papers on herd immunity or quoted by those speaking on herd immunity is a paper from 1971 by Fox, et.al. In this seminal paper, Fox states, "as defined in a medical dictionary, herd immunity is "the resistance of a group to attack by a disease to which a large proportion of the members are immune, thus lessening the likelihood of a patient with a disease coming into contact with a susceptible individual." This concept is directly applicable only to randomly mixing populations. However, truly random mixing can be assumed only for certain small closed populations and never occurs in open populations."(3) As is being pointed out in this paper, the concept of a "truly random mixing population" is an unlikely scenario and yet it is what is being assumed as the defacto starting position for the concept of herd immunity to be a successful proposition. The concept of herd immunity is essentially a mathematical construct being applied to a make believe population of randomly mixing individuals. The basics of the mathematical idea for herd immunity looks like this: "In general, the effective reproductive number (R) will be lower than the basic reproductive number (R 0), depending on the proportion (P) of the population who are immune to infection. Such immunity may be induced either by a previous infection with the agent (if such infection produced immunity) and/or by immunization with an effective vaccine. Simply, R = (1-P) * R0. Therefore, for infection elimination or eradication – i.e. to reduce R below 1, then P must be equal to at least (1-1/R 0). So, for example, if R0 = 5 then P must be at least (1-1/5) = 0.8. That is , 80% of the population must be immune, either through previous infection or vaccination. The value of P that reduces R to at most 1 is commonly called the "herd immunity threshold" – the level of population immunity that is necessary for the infection to be no longer self-sustaining in the population"(4) The paper from which this formula was taken goes on to present the following percentages, "Herd Immunity Thresholds (Approximate) for Infection

Elimination: Diphtheria 85%, Measles 83-94%, Mumps 75-86%, Pertussis 92-94%, Polio 80-86%, Rubella 83-85%, Smallpox 80-85%, Pandemic influenza (H1N1) ~40%."(4) These are the percentages that would need to be met in order to achieve this idea of herd immunity.

This idea of very specific percentages being necessary to achieve the concept of herd immunity is a common one that is seen on practically every website regarding vaccines and/or public health. The following quote is taken from the Columbia School of Public Health, "A large percentage of the population must be immune to the virus in some way in order to reach herd immunity. This threshold will vary depending on the disease—measles herd immunity requires 95% of the population to be immune, while polio requires 80%. In the case of COVID-19, health professionals estimate 70-90% of the population must be immune in order to achieve herd immunity."(5) And this quote is taken from the CDC, "The proportion of the population that has to be immune to provide this "herd immunity" varies according to the infectiousness of the agent. For poliomyelitis, that proportion is considered to be on the order of 80%, whereas for measles it exceeds 90%. Since 1981, vaccination levels in school entrants have been 95% or higher for diphtheria and tetanus toxoids and pertussis vaccine (DTP), polio vaccine, and measles vaccine. All states require vaccination for children attending licensed daycare centers and as a result such children have vaccination levels 90% or higher. Nonetheless, overall levels in preschool children have not been as high, as manifested by the resurgence of measles that occurred during 1989–1991, primarily affecting unvaccinated preschool-aged children. Levels in preschool-aged children have recently been raised to their currently high levels as a result of major efforts (and major infusions of resources) directed at this population. Nationwide, fewer than 1% of school entrants have medical, religious, or philosophic exemptions to mandatory vaccination. Seven states had more than 1% with exemptions in the 1997–1998 school year (Colorado, Michigan, Oregon, South Dakota, Utah, Washington, and West Virginia. Michigan had the highest level of exemption at 2.3%. However, in some communities, the levels of exemptors may be as high as 5%."(6) Notice that their own information is stating clearly that vaccination rates at the time of this quote were greater than 95% for DTP, polio and measles. A more recent assessment from the CDC of vaccine status, this one from 2017-2019, reported much the same. "National coverage by age 24 months was ≥90% for ≥3 doses of poliovirus vaccine, ≥3 doses of hepatitis B vaccine (HepB), and ≥1 dose of varicella vaccine (VAR); national coverage was ≥90% for ≥1 dose of measles, mumps, and rubella vaccine (MMR), although MMR coverage was <90% in 14 states. Only 1.2% of children had received no vaccinations by age 24 months."(7) Also notice that from the report done in 2007 to the one in 2019, the overall percentage of "unvaccinated" stayed right around 1%. To emphasize this point here again is the CDC, "The percentage of children who have received no vaccines has increased, reaching 1.3% for children born in 2015."(8)

According to research immunologist, Tetyana Obukhanych, PhD, "Herd immunity is a largely theoretical concept, yet for decades, it has furnished one of the key underpinnings for vaccine mandates in the United States. The public health establishment borrowed the herd immunity concept from pre-vaccine observations of natural disease outbreaks. Then, without any apparent supporting science, officials applied the concept to vaccination, using it not only to justify mass vaccination but to guilt-trip anyone objecting to the nation's increasingly onerous vaccine mandates. The truth is, diseases were already decreasing before their vaccines were introduced due to clean water & hygiene." Dr. Obukhanych goes on to illustrate some problems with the concept of herd immunity. "There are a number of other problems that make the theoretical concepts of vaccine efficacy & herd immunity highly imperfect in practice and, in fact, unachievable. These include:

- Secondary vaccine failure, defined as waning vaccine-induced immunity that no longer offers protection

- Mutation of the virus against which one is vaccinating, with the mutation plausibly triggered by the vaccine itself (vaccine researchers also allude to the problem of "genotype mismatch between the vaccine strain and the wild-type virus)

- Viral shedding that allows asymptomatic vaccinated individuals to transmit the vaccine strain of the illness

- Importation of illness due to travel

- Recurrent outbreaks of illness in vaccinated populations that, say Holland and Zachary, "scientists simply cannot explain"(9)

She further states that, "To prevent an outbreak, 70-95% of the population, according to very broad theoretical estimates, has to be truly immune – that is, resistant to viral infection, not just protected from developing the full range of symptoms that conform to the accepted clinical definition of the disease. However, 100% vaccination compliance can at best make only a quarter of the population become resistant to viral infection for more than a decade. This makes it apparent that stable herd immunity cannot be achieved via childhood vaccination in the long term regardless of the degree of vaccination compliance."(9)

According to the sources I have already quoted here, we have been over the 90% vaccinated compliance rate for decades. Once again here is the CDC and others on the percentages, "Vaccination coverage by the second birthday among children born during 2015–2016 remained high, with small increases in coverage with hepatitis A and B and influenza vaccines; only 1.3% of children received no vaccinations."(10) "As of 2017, around 91.5 percent of children in the U.S. aged 19 to 35 months had been vaccinated against measles, mumps and rubella (MMR)."(11) Remember that according to every "provax" source, if we hit the correct percentages, we should see these diseases ceasing to spread or even, by some estimates, eliminated. "Herd immunity can be thought of as a threshold level of immunity in the population above which a disease no longer spreads. For measles, the level of immunity needed to interrupt transmission is higher than the thresholds for almost all other vaccine preventable diseases—to prevent sustained spread of the measles virus, 92 to 94 % of the community must be protected."(12) "92-96% of children must be vaccinated to eliminate measles and pertussis, 84-88% to eliminate rubella and

88-92% to eliminate mumps in Western Europe and the United States..."(13) But are we actually seeing this? With decades of 90% plus vaccination rates we still see outbreaks of these very same diseases that the experts all agree should be controlled if not outright eliminated by the quoted vaccination rates. When we do see outbreaks of a "vaccine preventable disease" the immediate response from the media is that it is all on the shoulders of the unvaccinated. Those 1-2 percent of the population who are not supposed to be a factor according to their own mathematical calculations.

And what about these outbreaks? "We found 18 reports of measles outbreaks in very highly immunized school populations where 71% to 99.8% of students were immunized against measles. Despite these high rates of immunization, 30% to 100% (mean, 77%) of all measles cases in these outbreaks occurred in previously immunized students. In our hypothetical school model, after more than 95% of school children are immunized against measles, the majority of measles cases occur in appropriately immunized children."(14) "All cases had prior evidence of measles immunity. Symptoms were consistent with measles. Laboratory results indicated secondary immune responses. This is the first report of measles transmission from a twice vaccinated individual."(15) In 1989, "a large mumps outbreak occurred in Douglas County, Kansas. Of the 269 cases, 208 (77.3%) occurred among primary and secondary school students, of whom 203 (97.6%) had documentation of mumps vaccination."(16) In another mumps outbreak the researchers stated, "The overall attack rate is the highest reported to date (and to our knowledge) for a population demonstrating virtually complete mumps vaccine coverage."(17) And here yet another, "A chickenpox outbreak occurred in a school in which 97% of students without a prior history of chickenpox were vaccinated."(18) An interesting thing to note here is that the CDC is fully aware of some of these problems with the idea of herd immunity and their vaccines as they clearly state on their website, "Public health experts cannot rely on herd immunity to protect people from pertussis since: Pertussis spreads so easily, Vaccine protection decreases over time, Acellular pertussis vaccines may not prevent colonization (carrying the bacteria in your body without getting sick) or spread of the bacteria. (19) "The concept that a highly immune group of prepubertal children will prevent the spread of rubella in the rest of the community was shown by this epidemic not always to be valid."(20)

In fact, they are all well aware of some of the issues behind vaccine failures. "There are 2 major factors responsible for vaccine failures, the first is vaccine-related such as failures in vaccine attenuation, vaccination regimes or administration. The other is host-related, of which host genetics, immune status, age, health or nutritional status can be associated with primary or secondary vaccine failures."(21) "Primary vaccine failure could be defined as the failure to seroconvert or the failure to mount a protective immune response after vaccination despite seroconversion, whereas secondary vaccine failure is the gradual waning of immunity over time."(22) The CDC and the vaccine manufacturers both know that getting vaccinated does not mean that you can no longer catch the disease you have been vaccinated for nor does it mean that you can no longer spread said disease either. The topic of virus shedding from many of the vaccines is a topic with much research backing it.(23)(24)(25)(26) The recent Covid Pandemic and subsequent Covid vaccines have been a clear example of the failure of a vaccine to prevent the disease for which the vaccine was being mandated. The CDC was fully aware of the limitations and failures of their vaccine program, as noted in this report. "A total of 10,262 SARS-CoV-2 vaccine breakthrough infections had been reported from 46 U.S. states and territories as of April 30, 2021." In this same report they went on to talk about how that number of breakthrough infections was likely far higher. "...the number of reported COVID-19 vaccine breakthrough cases is likely a substantial undercount of all SARS-CoV-2 infections among fully vaccinated persons."(27) As usual the media did not discuss this aspect of the vaccine program. If we go back to the idea that a certain percentage of the population needs to be vaccinated in order for herd immunity to work, we can begin to see the problems inherent with the concept of herd immunity. First, while we can see clearly that children have been immunized for decades, at or close to the percentages stated to achieve herd immunity, adults are far from the numbers necessary. For adults over the age of 65, these are the following numbers: influenza vaccine = 69%, tetanus vaccine =

56.9%, pneumococcal vaccine = 63.6%, shingles vaccine = 34.2%(28), HPV vaccine = 16.5%(29), Tdap = 26.6%, Hepatitis A = 23.7%.(30) These numbers tend to be even lower for the ages between 19-65. Whether or not you know it, the Advisory Committee on Immunization Practices has a full set of vaccines recommended for adults. "Currently, the ACIP recommends immunizing adults against 15 infectious diseases, depending on age and varying risk criteria: influenza, diphtheria, tetanus, pertussis, varicella, human papillomavirus (HPV), zoster, mumps, measles, rubella, pneumococcal disease, meningococcal disease, hepatitis A, hepatitis B, and Haemophilus influenzae B."(31)

Many will assume that continuing vaccination among adults would not be necessary as the vast majority of adults have already been vaccinated as children and therefore should be immune to the various diseases. This however is an erroneous assumption. "Studies show vaccines for mumps, pertussis, meningococcal disease, and yellow fever also lose their effectiveness faster than official immunization recommendations suggest. "We simply don't know what the rules are to inducing long-lasting immunity," says Plotkin, who began to research vaccines in 1957. "For years, we were making vaccines without a really deep knowledge of immunology. Everything of course depends on immunologic memory, and we have not systematically measured it."(32) Stanley Plotkin, the person being quoted here, is widely considered an expert on the topic of vaccines. So the issues concerning adults and vaccination are: 1) Waning immunity from their childhood vaccines does not provide any lasting protection, 2) Adults never received many of the vaccines that are now being mandated to today's children so are therefore not "protected" from these diseases, and 3) The majority of adults have never kept current with any vaccine schedule, which therefore means no "boosting" of the original protection or no additional protection from new vaccines on the market.

With primary and secondary vaccine failures, false and waning immunity from the vaccines, viral mutations which the vaccines are not designed to affect, the importation of viruses from a global population and an adult population that is far below the percentages necessary to create herd immunity, the entire foundation upon which the concept of herd immunity is built begins to fall apart. The continued insistence for the creation of magical numbers that will protect all of mankind has already created in some minds, the idea that getting your vaccines is somehow a moral mandate. An excellent paper completed during the second year of the Covid pandemic illustrated this point very dramatically. The authors set out to show whether or not attitudes regarding Covid had become moralized. "When attitudes, including those regarding C19, are held with strong moral conviction, (known as moral mandates), they are perceived as objectively true and universally obligatory." "If these convictions are elevated to the status of a sacred value, merely questioning their authority can stimulate moral outrage and a desire to reaffirm one's moral convictions; a process known as moral cleansing." The researchers performed a study in America and one in New Zealand and their results showed confirmation of moralization in regards to questions of Covid-19. "People were more likely to accept social (shaming), health (illnesses and deaths resulting from statistical errors), and human rights costs (police abuse of power) when those costs resulted from Control-C19, than non-C19 efforts. Furthermore, when costs were incurred for non-C19 reasons (versus Control-C19 reasons), participants exhibited significantly greater moral outrage (all contexts), stronger punitive intentions towards responsible parties." This concept of vaccines being "elevated to a status of sacred value" has already been accomplished by the vaccine manufacturers and peddlers. The degree of moral outrage exhibited by so many people when the topic of vaccines is brought up is proof enough that this is true. Many individuals hold vaccines up to an almost Holy idea and anyone who goes against this "Holy idea" is immediately blasted as being against society. One of the biggest problems is when these beliefs are built upon information that is not as solid as it is being sold. Far too many people accept information at face value and build their belief system off of that information. This is true of many of the foundational points to which vaccines have been explained and sold to the general public of which herd immunity is one.

Point Number 13
Vaccine Ingredients

"Avoid food products containing ingredients that no ordinary human would keep in the pantry"
~Michael Pollan, American journalist and professor

How carefully do you look at the ingredients of the food you eat? What about the cleaning products in your home? How about pollution in the environment? What would you say is your level of concern regarding these things and other things that may impact your health? According to a survey by the Pew Research Center, "Some 44% of U.S. adults say they restrict or limit consumption of artificial sweeteners. A third (33%) say they limit artificial preservatives and 28% limit foods with artificial coloring." "The survey finds about half of Americans (49%) believe foods with GM (genetically modified) ingredients are worse for one's health" and "45% of Americans believe organic produce provides net benefits for health."(1) Another study by the IFIC (International Food Information Council) showed similar results, "IFC found slightly more than half (58%) of consumers strongly or somewhat strongly agree that they choose products with "clean ingredients whenever I grocery shop in person" and 56% strongly or somewhat agree that they avoid products with "chemically-sounding" ingredients. 48% said they avoid artificial preservatives at least some of the time." They went on to say, "66% of consumers surveyed say they strongly or somewhat agree that they pay more attention to ingredients on food and beverages than they did five years ago, and nearly two out of three say that ingredients have at least a moderate influence on their purchasing decisions."(2) And according to the website, *Statista*, "From 1999 to 2018, there has been a steady increase in worldwide sales of organic food. Worldwide organic food sales are now more than six times as large than they were in 1999, amounting to approximately 95 billion U.S. dollars in 2018."(3) *Statista* also reported that "In 2019, 43 percent of the respondents stated they were worried a "great deal" about air pollution."(4) These same basic results regarding attitudes are also seen when it comes to the cleaning products that we select. "Consumers are interested in cleaning up more than just their diet," concurs Kimberly Kawa, retail reporting analyst at Chicago-based SPINS, a provider of retail consumer insights, analytics and consulting for the natural, organic and specialty products industry. "Lifestyle and environment are also in focus, and natural cleaning products are a way to avoid exposure to undesirable constituents." Kawa goes on to note that sales of natural-positioned brands – a SPINS proprietary measure – have experienced a double-digit growth rate, while conventional products have seen only marginal growth."(5) This increased popularity in natural or "green" cleaning products has lead to a huge increase in revenue for companies that cater to this demand. "The global green cleaning products market accounted for US$ 3.9 billion in 2019 and is estimated to be US$ 11.6 billion by 2029 and is anticipated to register a CAGR (compound annual growth rate) of 11.8%."(6) So it seems that by all accounts there is a very large percentage of the population that cares deeply about what goes into their bodies and how these things may affect the overall health of their bodies. I wonder how many of these same people that care so deeply about how pesticides, artificial ingredients, or air and water pollution might impact their immediate and/or future health have ever considered (even for a moment) what they are allowing to be injected into their or their children's bodies through vaccines?

I am sure that for many, the ingredient list of vaccines would not change a thing for them. The idea that vaccines are necessary for the survival of mankind is so ingrained in the mentality of our society that the ingredient list of the vaccines that they are given would not even warrant thought. For the sake of argument, let's assume that , just like our food, air and water, what goes into our bodies makes a difference in our overall health. Let's assume that ingredients make a difference. Let's also assume that we should hold companies accountable for the ingredients that they place into items that are meant to go into our bodies. Many people likely think that vaccines are made up of portions of viruses for our bodies to have immune responses to and therefore build up a resistance to them. On the surface of things they are not wrong. That is the general premise. Vaccines do contain weakened, killed or parts of viruses or bacteria, however there is far more to the story than just this singular ingredient. It turns out that our bodies are so smart that when shown weakened, killed or parts of viruses or bacteria our body is not terribly concerned and therefore does not always promote a strong immune response. Vaccines therefore contain adjuvants, which are substances used to enhance the body's response to an antigen (some type of toxic or foreign substance that initiates an immune response). Vaccines will also usually contain other products to kill the virus or bacteria; stabilize the formula; and to sanitize it of contaminants. It is here that we start to see the myriad of ingredients that end up being injected into our children or ourselves.

If you were to ask the CDC or the pharmaceutical companies if there were anything amiss with any of the ingredients in the vaccines the answer would be a resounding "NO!" The patent answer is that the ingredients used in vaccines are perfectly safe and have stood the test of time. You can choose to believe this and simply trust that the CDC and pharmaceutical companies have your best interests as their primary concern and that they would never lie to you or mislead you (see Point 5) or you can look into this subject yourself and come to your own conclusions. Going that route, let's look at some of the ingredients that are commonly found in many of the vaccines being used today.

Common Ingredients found in vaccines:

- Aluminum: Used in (almost all) vaccines as an adjuvant. Many studies can be found which site the dangers or question the safety of aluminum in vaccines.(7,8,9,10) One study published in 2017 found that aluminum content was consistently high in brain tissue of those with autism.(11) They were not the only ones concerned about heavy metals showing up in autistic individuals, "Abnormal high levels of lead, mercury and aluminum, low level of zinc, were detected in the autistic featured group."(12) Another study from 2015 "suggests that aluminum-induced CRP (C-reactive Protein) may in part contribute to a pathophysiological state associated with a chronic systemic inflammation of the human vasculature."(13) And when the vaccine apologists tell you that there is nothing to be concerned about when it comes to aluminum in the vaccines, you can refer them to this study done in 2018, "Confirmation of their safety remains to be addressed and will only come from further research on their biological activities at injection sites and beyond. All ABAs (aluminum based adjuvants) currently in use in vaccination and subcutaneous immunotherapy require further validation of their safety."(14)

- Antibiotics: The most common antibiotics used in the production of vaccines are neomycin, polymyxin B, streptomycin and gentamicin. Antibiotics are used to prevent bacterial growth during the production process and during storage of the vaccines. Some known adverse effects of these particular antibiotics are: nephrotoxicity (kidney), ototoxicity (ear), neuromuscular blockade, cardiac effects and allergic reactions. The most common reactions are contact dermatitis and anaphylactic reactions.(15) Although only present in very small quantities their presence should still be factored in when we are looking at the entirety of what is being injected.

- Cell Culture Materials: Albumin is used as a growth medium when culturing the vaccine. It comes in a variety of forms: human serum albumin, bovine (cow) serum albumin, ovalbumin (egg), calf bovine (child cow) serum, fetal bovine serum (fetal cow). MRC-5 cellular proteins are derived from aborted human fetal material. Madin Darby canine kidney (mdck) cell protein comes from an adult female cocker spaniel that died in 1958. Baculovirus and Spodoptera frugiperda cell proteins (insect cell cultures), WI-38 human diploid lung fibroblasts from aborted human fetal material. Vero cells which are African Green Monkey kidney cells. Most vaccines contain combinations of the above materials.(16) The use of proteins in vaccines gives rise to concern over increasing food allergies in children as seen in the following quote form a paper written in 2015, "This combination of atopic children and food protein injection along with adjuvants, contributes to millions developing life threatening food allergies."(17) There is also research information discussing foreign DNA from fetal tissue used in vaccines in connection to autism: "Not only damaged human cells, but also healthy human cells can take up foreign DNA spontaneously. Foreign human DNA taken up by human cells will be transported into nuclei and be integrated into the host genome, which will cause phenotype change. Hence, residual human fetal DNA fragments in vaccines can be one of the causes of autism spectrum disorder in children through vaccination."(18)

- Formaldehyde: I for one do not want any of this injected into me until I am dead and gone. Formaldehyde is used in vaccines to kill viruses or inactivate toxins. One of the many concerns regarding vaccines has been the rise of asthma and a possible link with the increase in vaccines.(19,20,21) One study stated, "vaccination appears to increase the risk of allergies and related respiratory symptoms in children and adolescents."(22) One possible link is formaldehyde, "The results suggest that domestic exposure to formaldehyde increases the risk of childhood asthma."(23) A separate study showed similar findings, "An association between exposure to formaldehyde and sensitization to common aeroallergens has been suggested from animal trials."(24) A paper from the EPA explained formaldehydes toxic effects, "Exposure of experimental animals to formaldehyde results in its rapid metabolic incorporation into DNA, RNA, and proteins, demonstrating that exogenous formaldehyde mixes readily with the endogenous pool and in the covalent binding of formaldehyde to these macromolecules. The covalent reactions of formaldehyde with macromolecules are generally accepted as the fundamental causes of its toxic effects."(25)

- Monosodium Glutamate (MSG): MSG is used as a stabilizer to protect vaccines from a variety of things such as heat, light and acidity. While many medical sites debunk the idea that MSG is harmful, not everyone is in agreement with that notion. "Different studies have hinted at possible toxic effects related to this popular food-additive. These toxic effects include CNS disorder, obesity, disruptions in adipose tissue physiology, hepatic damage, CRS and reproductive malfunctions. These threats might have hitherto been underestimated."(26) Another study published in 2020, dismissed some of the notions regarding MSG while tacking on this little gem, "Another issue that would benefit from further studies is the impact of dietary MSG on fetal development. Preclinical studies indicated behavioral changes in the rats born from mothers exposed to MSG, but due to the design of these studies, it is hard to establish their relevance for human prenatal exposure."(27) Very interesting.

- Polysorbate 80: Used in vaccines as a stabilizer. This is one of the most interesting components to me and potentially the most deadly. A multitude of websites will profess the safety of polysorbate 80 even mentioning the myriad of food products it is in while discussing how safe it is. Contrast this with the published research articles out there and you begin to wonder where the "safety" of this product is coming from. A paper published in 2017 investigated the safety of polysorbate 80. Their conclusion, "PSM, the theoretical target product of polysorbate 80, was proved to possess acute toxicity on zebrafish [Zebrafish are considered as an ideal candidate for acute toxicity evaluation of complicated mixtures because it possesses genes highly homologous to human genes and signal transduction pathways similar to humans] among all the isolated components, indicating that (1) pharmaceutical excipients including complicated mixtures as polysorbate 80 have potential risks and the present quality standards are not sufficient for their quality control, and (2) the optimal component ratio of pharmaceutical excipients and their toxicity should be further investigated in detail."(27) What makes polysorbate 80 really dangerous when it comes to being a component of vaccines is its ability to adversely affect the blood-brain barrier. The blood-brain barrier protects our brain by creating a highly selective barrier that does not allow certain things from gaining access to the brain (such as bacteria, toxins and foreign substances).(29,30,31,32,33,34) So take this ability to allow access to the brain and add aluminum, thimerosal, food proteins and more. Are you beginning to see the picture? Add to this already horrible information that research shows that some individuals also can have serious allergic reactions to polysorbate 80.(35)

- Thimerosal: Used as a preservative in vaccines. Thimerosal has been used widely in vaccine production since the 1930's. It was removed from most vaccines in the U.S. in 2001. It is still used in the seasonal flu vaccines (there are non-thimerosal versions if you ask for them). Thimerosal is still widely used in vaccines outside of the U.S. (36) Of all ingredients found in vaccines, none has been talked about more than thimerosal. Although the vaccine defenders would love to make you think thimerosal has been thoroughly investigated and that it has been proven safe and proven to have no involvement in autism, the truth is not as clean and clear as they would have you believe. The research has never stated that thimerosal is harmless nor has it actually been "proven to have no correlation with the development of autism. See Point 8 and Point 11 for more on research regarding thimerosal. This paper published in 2012 had this to say about thimerosal, "Our data showed an effect of organic mercury on the viability of Jurkat T cells, suggesting a possible toxic effect of these compounds of mercury in vivo." (37) This study from 2011 said this, "Thimerosal at concentrations relevant for infants' exposure (in vaccines) is toxic to cultured human-brain cells and to laboratory animals." (38) This study from 2009 showed an increased correlation between thimerosal exposure and the male gender in mice, "the first report of gender-selective toxicity of thimerosal and indicate that any future studies of thimerosal toxicity should take into consideration gender-specific differences." (39) If you have followed autism information at all you will know that boys are more affected than girls. Thimerosal is the perfect example of how those who vigorously defend vaccines work very hard to get you to believe something that is simply not true.

When the subject of vaccine injuries comes up or the cause of autism comes up, those that defend vaccines say that it is a proven fact that vaccines are safe and that they do not cause autism. The problem with these statements is that they are built on half truths and supposition. To say that vaccines do not cause autism based on a handful of studies of thimerosal is stretching things to the point of breaking. As I mentioned back in Point Ten, there may have been studies done on individual vaccines however, there has never been a study done on all of the vaccines as a group entity. Recognizing that the vaccine schedule as a whole with all of the combinations of viruses and ingredients combined is vastly different than looking at a singular vaccine is paramount to understanding the effects that may be occurring to our children as a result. Nothing exists in a vacuum and the vaccines should not be looked at as individual entities with no cross over consequences. The proper research has not and is not being done to truly see what affects the vaccine schedule as a whole may be causing nor are the individual and combined effects of the ingredients really being looked at either. When combined as a cocktail, the ingredients and the number of vaccines as a whole are potentially causing a great number of concerning situations. That no one in authority seems to be taking this seriously is alarming.

Point Number 14
Chicken Pox and Shingles

"Cause and effect are two sides of one fact."
~ Ralph Waldo Emerson, American essayist

The one idea that it seems everyone in favor of vaccines will argue, is that they are 100% necessary and that the long term benefits are worth it. To show how this idea does not necessarily hold up under scrutiny for all of the vaccines in the childhood schedule, you need look no further than the chickenpox vaccine. The chickenpox vaccine came onto the market in 1995. This was part of the new vaccine surge that came after the pharmaceutical companies became free and clear from liability for their products. During my research into this subject, every expert I read agreed that chicken pox is a mild and limiting disease that the vast majority of children move through with no harm done to them. Not only do the vast majority of children come away from a chicken pox infection with no serious harm, they also come away from it with immunity and protection, especially from the secondary infection known as shingles. According to the CDC, "In healthy children, varicella is generally mild, with an itchy rash, malaise, and temperature up to 102°F for 2 to 3 days. In otherwise healthy people, a second occurrence of varicella is uncommon. As with other viral infections, re-exposure to natural (wild-type) varicella may lead to re-infection that boosts antibody titers without causing illness or detectable viremia."(1) In fact, according to the CDC's own information, the risk of death from chicken pox prior to the introduction of the vaccine was .00375. Looking at this information it is hard to understand why chicken pox was considered a threat worthy of vaccination.

Whereas chicken pox is typically very mild and rarely serious, its secondary infection, shingles, can be more painful and potentially more deadly especially in older individuals. After an initial infection by chicken pox, the virus can lie dormant in neural tissue near the spinal cord and brain. The virus may be "awakened" years later when age, disease, stress or something else weakens the immune system sufficiently to allow it to re-emerge. In fact, "complications from shingles in the elderly can lead to serious, long-term health problems. They range from bacterial skin infections that can cause scarring and necrotizing fasciitis to hearing and vision loss, encephalitis, transverse myelitis, peripheral motor neuropathy, and postherpetic neuralgia (PHN)." (2) It is actually repeated exposure to the chickenpox virus throughout life that keeps the virus from re-emerging as shingles. It is also why "some countries have worried that chickenpox vaccinations might inadvertently increase the number of shingles cases." (3) This is a situation that science has already theorized as is evidenced by this quote, "since varicella is commonly a benign disease in childhood, a rise in the incidence of herpes zoster in older people could occur, due to lack of boosting throughout life".(4)

There are many research papers that discuss the very real situation of the chickenpox vaccine leading to increases in herpes zoster infection, or shingles, later in life. From a paper written back in 1999 the authors expressed their concern by mentioning, "two possible dangers of an extensive varicella vaccination program are more varicella (chickenpox) cases in adults, when the complication rates are higher, and an increase in cases of zoster (shingles)."(5) In another study that looked at the rates of varicella infection and herpes zoster infection in the state of Massachusetts over the time period between 1998 and 2003, the authors found that "as varicella vaccine coverage in children increased, the incidence of varicella decreased and the occurrence of herpes zoster increased." In fact the increase in cases of herpes zoster in older individuals was between 41-161 percent!(6) Another study published in 2002 mentioned, "recent evidence suggests that an increase in zoster incidence appears likely, and the more effective vaccination is at preventing varicella, the larger the increase in zoster incidence."(7) Yet another paper written in 2009, showed an "unexplained" "incidence of herpes zoster among 10- to 19-year-olds... by 63%" after the initiation of the chicken pox vaccination program.(8)

Not every nation has felt the same as the U.S. does when it comes to establishing a mandatory vaccine for chickenpox. "The introduction of mass vaccination against Varicella-Zoster-Virus (VZV) is being delayed in many European countries because of, among other factors, the possibility of a large increase in Herpes Zoster (HZ) incidence in the first decades after the initiation of vaccination, due to the expected decline of the boosting of Cell Mediated Immunity caused by the reduced varicella circulation."(9) The UK had a "unique" outlook when it came to this vaccine as well. "Chickenpox in the United Kingdom, where vaccination is not undertaken, has had a stable epidemiology for decades and is a routine childhood illness. Because of vaccination, chickenpox is now a rarity in the USA. In the UK vaccination is not done because introduction of a routine childhood vaccination might drive up the age at which those who are non-immune get the illness (chickenpox tends to be more severe the older you are), and the incidence of shingles may increase. The United Kingdom is waiting to see what happens in countries where vaccination is routine. There is a general principle that it is best to acquire childhood illnesses (including, chickenpox, measles, and glandular fever) in childhood."(10) A "general principle that it is best to acquire childhood illnesses." What a novel concept. It is no wonder that so many in Europe were so highly skeptical regarding the vaccination program when studies, like this one done in Germany, showed a doubling of herpes zoster infection after the initiation of the vaccination program. (11)

Gary S. Goldman, Ph.D., who served for eight years as a Research Analyst with the Varicella Active Surveillance Project conducted by the Los Angeles County Department of Health Services (LACDHS) (a project funded by the CDC), has been a widely published and highly vocal opponent of the CDC's chicken pox Gary S. Goldman, Ph.D., who served for eight years as a Research Analyst with the Varicella Active Surveillance Project conducted by the Los Angeles County Department of Health Services (LACDHS) (a project funded by theCDC), has been a widely published and highly vocal opponent of the CDC's chicken pox chickenpox. Goldman's analysis in *International Journal of Toxicology (IJT)* indicates that effectiveness of the chickenpox vaccine itself is also dependent on natural boosting, so that as chickenpox declines, so does the effectiveness of the vaccine. "The principal reason that vaccinees in Japan maintained high levels of immunity 20 years following vaccination was that only 1 in 5 (or 20%) of Japanese children were vaccinated," he said. "So those vaccinated received immunologic boosting from contact with children with natural chickenpox. But the universal varicella vaccination program in the U.S. will nearly eradicate this natural boosting mechanism and will leave our population vulnerable to shingles epidemics."(12) "Goldman points out that during a 50-year time span, there would be an estimated additional 14.6 million (42%) shingles cases among adults aged less than 50 years, presenting society with a substantial additional medical cost burden of $4.1 billion. This translates into $80 million annually, utilizing an estimated mean healthcare provider cost of $280 per shingles case."(12) Goldman eventually left his work with the CDC when after data was manipulated to "conceal unwanted outcomes that supported an immunologically-mediated link between varicella and herpes zoster (HZ) epidemiology."(13) In a paper published in the *Annals of Clinical Pathology*, Goldman wrote: "The CDC mainly published selective studies and manipulated findings to support universal varicella vaccination and aggressively blocked the Research Analyst's (Goldman's) attempt to publish deleterious trends or outcomes (e.g., declining vaccine efficacy, increasing HZ incidence rates, etc.), prompting his resignation in protest against what he perceived was research fraud. His (Goldman's) letter of resignation stated, "When research data concerning a vaccine used in human populations is being suppressed and/or misrepresented, this is very disturbing and goes against all scientific norms and compromises professional ethics."(13) If you want to read a report that speaks to the type of "cover-ups," fraud and abuse in the scientific system that I have been alluding to throughout this book, this paper is a perfect example.

A very recent study (2021) illustrated the absence of economic benefit with the chickenpox vaccine program, just as Goldman had already pointed out. In this study, the authors "undertook a cost-utility analysis of the chickenpox vaccination from both a publicly funded healthcare payer and societal perspective" in Canada.(14) The study looked at three different scenarios over a 175 year period. Scenario one was no vaccination while scenarios two and three were different variations of vaccination programs. Their results: "When we incorporated the effect of shingles into our analysis, we found that vaccination was cost-ineffective from the healthcare perspective. Again, these results were consistent with previous cost-effectiveness studies, which demonstrated that the increased severity of shingles infection and the costs associated with treatment and productivity loss generally outweighed the benefits of reducing chickenpox infection."(14)

Not only do we have a vaccination that by all standards was not even necessary to begin with, but it is a vaccination that is actually creating a situation that is potentially more deadly than the disease for which it is attempting to help. By increasing the risks of shingles in older individuals, this vaccine is possibly creating a far more harmful situation. Add to this the lack of cost benefit and you might think this would be enough to have folks wondering, "Why did we agree to this?" We can also add to this list of reasons why this vaccine should not even be on a list of mandatory vaccines, the question of its effectiveness and its safety. As with other vaccines, the chickenpox vaccine does have a high risk of "breakthrough" cases. (Breakthrough cases being cases where people still get the disease for which they were vaccinated for.) According to the CDC, "25% to 30% of people vaccinated with one dose (of the chickenpox vaccine) who get breakthrough varicella will have clinical features similar to unvaccinated people with varicella. People with breakthrough varicella with 50 or more lesions were just as contagious as unvaccinated people with the disease."(1) As for the varicella vaccine's safety...the only source we have for assessing this is VAERS. I have already discussed the accuracy and effectiveness of VAERS in previous Points. The only item I shall mention as a reminder is that according to a Harvard study less than 1% of adverse events are actually reported to VAERS.(15) With this information in mind, "VAERS received 6,574 case reports of adverse events in recipients of varicella vaccine, a rate of 67.5 reports per 100,000 doses sold.

Approximately 4% of reports described serious adverse events, including 14 deaths. Admitting that underreporting made the figures "highly variable fractions of actual event numbers," the authors revealed that approximately 4 percent of cases (about 1 in 33,000 doses) were serious."(16) When you consider that this vaccination is not truly necessary for the health and protection of our children, any injuries at all from this vaccine are totally unacceptable. And, when you consider that the adverse events mentioned above could very well be only 1% of the actual number of adverse events out there, then we are now entering an area where we should be questioning the validity of the usage of this vaccine. At the very least, to be able to defend the usage of a given vaccine, you should be able to show two clear things: the vaccine is necessary to save lives and it does no harm. I am not sure that this can be said when it comes to the varicella vaccine.

How is a vaccine allowed to (not only) come on to the market, but also get placed onto the list of mandatory vaccines when: #1 The virus it is designed for is not a realistic threat to those that get it, #2 Those that get the virus receive life long immunity, #3 The vaccine may place millions at risk of a far more threatening condition (shingles), #4 The vaccine has a high breakthrough case percentage (25-30%), #5 The vaccine has been shown to be less cost effective than natural immunity, and #6 The vaccine has a potentially far greater risk to health than the actual virus did? Being that this vaccine came about in 1995 soon after the pharmaceutical companies were given freedom from liability, your conspiracy would be as good as mine. I can tell you that this vaccine has been a gold mine for Merck (the manufacturer of Varivax). An article from 2016 listed Varivax as the fourth most successful vaccine in pharmaceutical history; profiting Merck 1.5 billion dollars in 2015 alone.(17) Add to this the fact that Merck had also created the first vaccine for shingles. Remember that tons of available evidence showed that the introduction of a varicella vaccine would likely lead to a large increase in the number of shingles cases. Zostavax, Merck's shingles vaccine, brought in over 685 million in 2016, but of course that was before the vaccine started injuring and killing people.(18) By the way, Gardasil's shingles vaccine, Shingrix, is expected to bring in over 1.37 billion a year in 2022. Does any of this prove that all of this is entirely motivated by money? Of course it does not, however, as the old expression says, money talks. The financial motivations behind vaccines in general from both the pharmaceutical industry side and the government side make it difficult to see how something like the varicella vaccine was ever allowed to become a mandatory vaccination unless there was some incentive to move it forward to where it is today. Not only did we get a vaccine for chickenpox but we also got one for shingles. Two for the price of one. And the pharmaceutical companies win yet again.

Point Number Fifteen
Risks versus Benefits

"Information is power. Think for yourself. CAUTION: proper use of the brain is not endorsed by federal governments nor huge corporations involved in serious financial profit from a brainwashed and enslaved population. Mild discomfort may occur as confusing independent thought challenges popular views of the world."
~Timothy Leary

The importance of making informed, educated decisions is always important, but even more so when the issue is something that will impact your health and your child's health. Having access to as much information and evidence as you can is paramount towards making the best decisions you can for you and your family. Unfortunately, when it comes to vaccination the individual is rarely given the honest and unbiased information they need to make this incredibly important decision. The vaccine apologists would certainly argue this point by saying that, by law, pediatricians must give out Vaccine Information Statements (VIS) to the parents prior to their children getting their vaccinations. This is, of course, a technically accurate statement, however the information presented on the VIS handouts is not an honest or unbiased representation of the research or information that is necessary for a person to truly make an informed decision. (1) Not only are the handouts completely slanted in favor of getting the vaccines, but not all pediatricians are even giving out this biased material to every parent.

The ability to access unbiased, multidirectional, non-agenda oriented information has been further impeded by the various social media platforms. Even getting access to the information that is found in this book was made more challenging due to the updated algorithm changes on Google, Youtube and other platforms. When I first started gathering research on vaccines back in the early 2000's, all you needed to do was type what you were looking for in the search bar and you would be rewarded with a list of information that had not been cultivated by the vaccine apologists. Now if you type anything regarding vaccines you will get a thoroughly edited version of information courtesy of the vaccine agenda. Any information that goes against the narrative is buried and obfuscated. You can still find the information but you need to know where and how to look for it to find it. This means that the average individual will not find it. Certainly parents who do a cursory search for information will only end up seeing the information that the CDC and pharmaceutical companies want you to find. Adding to all of this is the seemingly complete control of all basic media now when it comes to the messaging around anything related to vaccines. The near complete blackout of any information that questions the vaccine imperative is astounding and frankly scary. The deck is certainly stacked against anyone who casually goes looking for any vaccine information that is contrary to what the government and pharmaceutical companies want everyone to know.

One of the most important points of information to understand when choosing any medical intervention, is the risks of the intervention (or of not choosing said intervention) versus the benefits of the intervention. As previously mentioned, the information that is given out to those looking into vaccination for themselves or their children gives an incredibly slanted view of the risks versus benefits. Anyone who only sees the information given to them by the typical pediatrician or from a cursory search on Google will come away with the view point that to not vaccinate is crazy or worse, suicide/murder. Getting access to reliable information about risks versus benefits is difficult. In this Point I am going to choose a sampling of the vaccines to attempt to show you the risks of the particular virus versus the risk of the vaccine for that virus. The gold standard for this information was written in 1996 and last updated in 2002 by Randall Neustaedter, OMD and is called *The Vaccine Guide*. In this excellent book, Dr. Neustaedter does a very thorough job of breaking down this information for all of the vaccines that were being given at the time the book was last updated. This was one of the first vaccine books I read when I began seriously looking into this subject. So let's take a look at some of the diseases and their related vaccines.

The Flu Vaccine

According to the VIS for Flu, it is more dangerous for "infants and young children, people 65 years and older, pregnant people, and people with certain health conditions or a weakened immune system." So, of course, accordingly, the CDC "recommends everyone 6 months and older get vaccinated every flu season." (2) Essentially this means everyone should get this vaccine according to the CDC. If the CDC feels that everyone must get this vaccine, it follows that the virus associated with it must be a really nasty bugger to warrant such protection against it.

The World Health Organization states that the IFR of influenza is between .029 - .065. (3) Meaning that among all individuals who become infected with influenza less than 1% of these individuals will die from the flu. Put another way, if you catch the flu you have about a 99.5% chance (or greater) to survive it. Put another way, not so dire. As per the VIS, the common response to catching the flu is "fever and chills, sore throat, muscle aches, fatigue, cough, headache, and runny or stuffy nose." (2) Is it fun to catch the flu? No, to put it frankly, it sucks, but does this constitute a necessity for vaccination? For the answer to this question we need to also look at the risks of taking the vaccine.

The VIS states that the most common adverse reactions are "soreness, redness, and swelling where the shot is given, fever, muscle aches, and headache." If given at the same time as the DTaP (very common if a child) it can also cause seizures. It also acknowledges the remote chance of "a severe allergic reaction, other serious injury, or death." Also mentioned is the "very small increased risk of Guillain-Barré Syndrome (GBS)." (2) According to a study done back in 1976, the overall rate of GBS was "significantly higher among vaccine recipients than in nonrecipients." (4) Then in 1991, another study was done to reassess this data regarding GBS which reconfirmed the risks stating that there was an "increased risk of developing Guillain-Barré syndrome during the 6 weeks following vaccination in adults." (5) I found another study done in 2009 that concluded that "The highest number of GBS cases was observed in subjects receiving influenza vaccine followed by hepatitis B vaccine." (6) Lifetime complications from GBS can include: being unable to walk without assistance, weakness in arms,legs and face, balance and coordination problems, numbness/pain and extreme tiredness. The CDC may proclaim the risk of getting GBS as "very small," but the risk of serious harm from the virus is also very small and the typical person will get over the flu with zero complications, not so much with GBS.

The CDC recommends the flu vaccine for pregnant women (7), even though pregnant women are very rarely (6%) part of the research trials for vaccines. (8, 9, 10) The reality is the CDC (and no one else) really understands the harmful effect vaccines may have on pregnant women. While limited, studies have already pointed out the increased risk of spontaneous abortion with vaccination. (11,12,13) The fact is we really do not understand the longer term consequences of vaccination on pregnant women (or their unborn child) as the studies have simply not been done. As for the other high risk group being asked to get the flu shot seasonally, the elderly, the benefit of vaccination may be over rated according to some researchers. So said the authors of a research article printed in the *Archives of Internal Medicine*, "we conclude that observational studies substantially overestimate vaccination benefit [among the elderly]." (14) Another study out of the University of Toronto found that "vaccination was linked with a 6% reduction in all-cause mortality during flu seasons, but this difference was not statistically significant." Epidemiologists M. Alan Brookhart, PhD, and Leah McGrath, MS, commented on this study saying that "the findings are consistent with three recent US studies suggesting that the life-saving benefits of flu vaccine in the elderly are small." (15) One last study to consider, found that "respiratory infections were caused mostly by pathogens other than influenza virus during the influenza period documented nationally. This highlights the role of coronaviruses, respiratory syncytial virus, and unidentified agents in the elderly, and questions the assumptions made in American on the impact of influenza and the value of influenza vaccines." (16)

The flu vaccine hovers around a 40% effectiveness on average (some years as low as 10% or as much as 60%). (17) You have no way of knowing which level of effectiveness your vaccine will be however, which begs the question as to whether or not the risks associated with the vaccine will be worth the less than 50% effectiveness of the shot. And, by the way, the flu vaccine is one of the only vaccines that still utilizes thimerosal, the mercury preservative that has been removed from most vaccines due to questions of safety.

Summary: The seasonal flu has an incidence of fatality of less than 1%. The flu vaccine contains thimerosal and has been linked to increased risks of Guillain-Barré Syndrome. The vaccine's seasonal effectiveness is only around 40%.

The Chickenpox Vaccine

It has long been known that varicella (chickenpox) is a very benign disease. In an article in the *British Medical Journal* dated 1961, the authors refer to varicella as "a highly infectious disease of children, usually mild in nature, without complications or sequelae." (18) Jump ahead to another article written in the journal Pediatrics in 1986 and here the authors essentially state the same thing, "varicella has long been considered a benign, inevitable disease of childhood." They continue stating, "complications are generally mild and rarely severe, and virtually every individual is infected by adulthood." (19) However, if you were to read the VIS for varicella you may likely come away with a far more foreboding outlook on this disease. Within the first two paragraphs of the VIS it does have the four words that state, "Chickenpox is usually mild" however every other word within these two paragraphs attempts to present varicella as a very scary, major illness that can lead to brain issues and death. (20) Instead of focusing on the reality that this disease is rarely ever serious for the vast majority of people who contract it, they instead focus on emphasizing the very rare incidences of severity.

The VIS mentions the "rare" adverse reactions from the vaccine such as: pneumonia, infection of the brain and/ or spinal cord covering, or seizures that are often associated with fever. The VIS also makes the statement that for "people with serious immune system problems, this vaccine may cause an infection that may be life-threatening." This, by the way, is the same population of people (immunocompromised) that the VIS points out are at risk for the more serious problems associated with contracting the virus and therefore should be getting the vaccine. The VIS also mentions that the vaccination can lead to a rash that can then spread chicken pox to other individuals and that the vaccination can still result in shingles years later (although less likely than natural infection according to the VIS).

This is a nice segway into what is likely the larger concern over the chickenpox vaccination, which is the rise in shingles. When a person contracts chickenpox, the body fights off the virus but does not actually completely destroy or get rid of the virus from the person's system. Instead, the virus retreats to the ganglia near the spinal cord where it lies dormant until a stressor may reactivate it in some people. This is what we then refer to as shingles. The prevailing theory is that repeat exposures to the varicella virus helps to keep the virus from reemerging and creating shingles. The success of the chickenpox vaccine however, has reduced overall exposure rates to varicella and therefore has led to the recent explosion in shingles cases. (21,22,23) In essence, we have traded chickenpox for shingles. Chickenpox, which I have already shown to be widely agreed upon as a benign disease of childhood, in exchange for shingles, a condition that can lead to much more serious issues in adults. Shingles has a much higher probability of causing serious issues, such as: loss of vision, debilitating pain, disseminated zoster, post-herpetic neuralgia, and other complications. (24) Of course, the brilliant minds that brought you the chickenpox vaccine have now brought you the shingles vaccine. One vaccine to help counteract the problems created by a different vaccine.

<u>Summary</u>: Chickenpox is a very mild childhood disease with incredibly low complications for the majority of children. The vaccine has side-effects that are higher or equal to any issues one may get from the actual virus. The usage of this vaccine has most likely led to the increase of a more serious condition (shingles).

The Pertussis (Whooping Cough) Vaccine

Pertussis is one of many diseases that the vaccine apologists love to cite as proof of how vaccination has saved everyone. In Point 2, I discussed the falsity of this idea that the vaccines are the saviors of mankind and that disease rates were fast declining well before the introduction of the vaccines. I will reiterate that I am not saying that vaccines have made no difference to disease rates, but to hold them up in divine light as saviors is not a true story to sell the public. Below is another graph taken from the book Dissolving Illusions that clearly illustrates the sharp decline that pertussis was taking long before the vaccines were introduced.

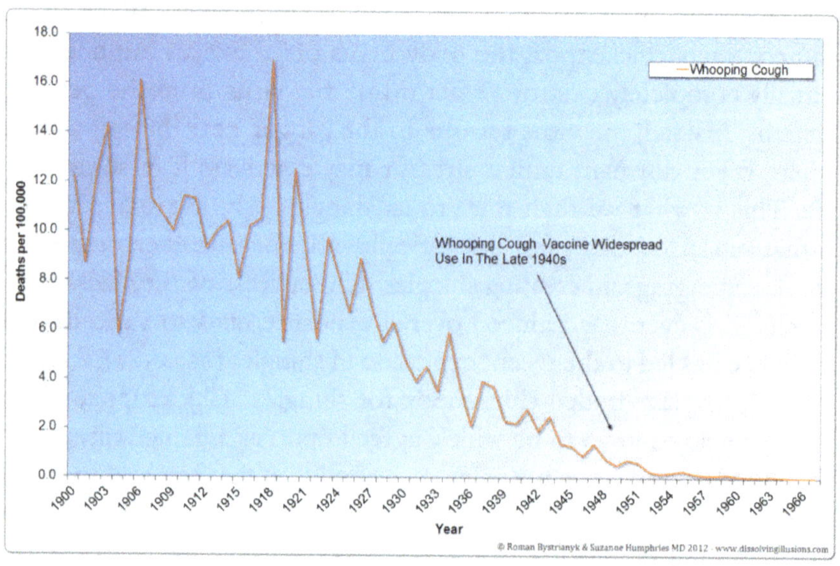

It would also be difficult to make the idea stick that pertussis vaccines would have had a dramatic effect on the number of cases knowing how poorly the vaccines work in any long term capacity. (25, 26) The number of reported outbreaks from mostly or even fully vaccinated populations clearly shows the limited or poor effect of these vaccines. (27, 28, 29, 30, 31) Not only are the outbreaks occurring in highly vaccinated populations but a study done in 2020 stated that asymptomatic (vaccinated) persons may be responsible for the spread of pertussis, "Our results demonstrate a high prevalence of subclinical infection in household contacts of pertussis cases, which may play asubstantial role in the ongoing transmission of disease." (32) Despite the clear evidence of the vaccine's failures, the story headlines still place all blame for any outbreaks on the 2% of Americans that choose not to vaccinate.

Pertussis can have serious consequences such as pneumonia, convulsions, brain damage, or death. This is far more serious in babies and the very young (under one year). The vaccine has its own issues however that need to be considered before making a decision. The VIS for DTaP only states the usual adverse reactions that are typically shown on all of the VIS: "Soreness or swelling where the shot was given, fever, fussiness, feeling tired, loss of appetite, and vomiting." The only "serious reactions" mentioned are "seizures, non-stop crying for 3 hours or more, or high fever (over 105°F)." (33) A study that was performed back in 1985 had a much different view of the pertussis vaccine that actually stated, "the risk of pertussis vaccine...exceeded those of whooping cough." (34) This same study even went a step further and shot down one of the most common arguments for needing to be vaccinated, herd immunity, by stating "There was no evidence of a herd immunity sufficient to protect infants below age for vaccination." A study performed in 1977 illustrated far more serious consequences from taking the vaccine, "16 cases of neurological disease and/or death shortly after pertussis immunization are reported. Eight patients had convulsions, six with ensuing permanent defects. Severe polymyositis was observed in one case. Five infants died 12 h to 4 days after vaccination: two after acute encephalopathy and three in the form of a sudden unexpected death (SID)." (35) This same study also pointed out that this was most likely a larger problem by stating that "It is concluded that only a minor proportion of possible complications is presently reported to the health authorities." And yet another study performed around the same time period (1977) showed "Twenty cases of acute neurological complications occurring within 7 days of pertussis immunization are reported." (36) Another paper published in 2017, looked at the introduction of the DTP vaccine in Guinea-Bissau in the early 1980s and found that the DTP vaccine "was associated with increased mortality." (37) While that paper looked backwards, in another paper published in 2017 an Israeli MD discussed a patient withacute disseminated encephalomyelitis (ADEM) and the possibility that it stemmed from the pertussis vaccination (38). In this paper the doctor discusses ADEM as a "post-vaccination phenomenon." This is backed up by a paper published in 2008 that stated, "Post-vaccination ADEM has been associated with several vaccines such as rabies, diphtheria-tetanus-polio, smallpox, measles, mumps, rubella, Japanese B encephalitis, pertussis, influenza, hepatitis B, and the Hog vaccine." (39)

Summary: Pertussis can have severe results with mostly very young children and babies. Both the whole-cell and acellular versions of the pertussis vaccine can cause encephalitis, seizures, brain damage and death. The vaccine has a limited efficacy and may even spread the virus

The Hepatitis B Vaccine

For the last sampling for this particular discussion, I chose the Hepatitis B vaccine. The Hep B vaccine first became commercially available in 1982. The original design was to give this to high risk individuals such as healthcare workers (less than 5% of cases), intravenous drug users, and people with multiple sexual partners. People who had an actual risk of possibly contracting hepatitis B. This turned out to be a failed plan because getting these groups to take the vaccine proved far too difficult. (40) So, the game plan was altered and the decision was made to begin giving the Hep B vaccine to infants as a part of the vaccine schedule for all children.

Infections from hepatitis B virus are "transmitted when blood, semen, or another body fluid from a person infected with HBV enters the body of someone who is not infected. This can happen through sexual contact; sharing needles, syringes, or other drug-injection equipment; or from mother to baby at birth." (41) According to Health and Human Services, "in the United States, in 2018, injection drug use was the most common risk factor reported among people with an acute HBV infection, followed by having multiple sex partners." (41) The only way that newborns are at risk for HBV infection is from mother-to-child transmission. The primary population of women at risk forHBV infection (and therefore able to pass HBV on to their fetus) are drug addicts and sex-workers. (42) This limited population means that the vast majority of infants have no real risk of exposure to HBV whatsoever. There have long been measures in place to screen and test for HBV infection in pregnant women and preventative measures to care for infants infected from their mothers. With the steps that were already in place for high risk populations it seems entirely unnecessary to add another vaccination to infants for a virus they have absolutely no risk for acquiring.

Since the vast majority of newborns have no risk for exposure to the Hep B virus, any risks associated with the vaccine would completely nullify any reasons for injecting said vaccination into infants. Multiple studies involving mice injected with the Hep B vaccine have shown a number of alarming results. Liver damage, gastrointestinal disease and even neurobehavioral problems were shown in these various animal studies. (43,44,45,46,47,48) Other studies have reported autoimmune manifestations such as rheumatoid arthritis, reactive arthritis, vasculitis, encephalitis, neuropathy, and thrombocytopenia. (49) But let's not stop there, yet more studies have associated the Hep B vaccine to neuromuscular disorders, acute disseminated encephalomyelitis (ADEM), chronic fatigue syndrome, fibromyalgia and more. (50,51,52,53) Another concern involving this vaccine is the incidence of Guillain-Barré syndrome (GBS). As one study commented, "the highest number (n = 632) of GBS cases was observed in subjects receiving influenza vaccine followed by hepatitis B vaccine." (54) The incredibly high number of associated issues following vaccination with Hep B is alarming. This is made especially so as this vaccine is wholly unnecessary.

<u>Summary</u>: Infection with HBV occurs almost exclusively in drug addicts and sex workers. Infants are typically only at risk if their mother has HBV infection at the time of birth. Measures are already in place to test pregnant women for HBV infection and to treat the infants of infected mothers. The HBV vaccine has a high incidence of possible side-effects and complications.

Many people do not realize that when it comes to making the decision to vaccinate your children, the CDC's childhood schedule is only one option. You can choose to fully vaccinate according to the schedule. You can choose to completely avoid all vaccines (there are exemptions). You can also choose an alternative schedule. The idea that you have to vaccinate according to the CDC's full schedule is not entirely true. A parent can choose to delay the schedule or choose to not receive particular vaccines. While many pediatricians may insist that a parent follow the complete schedule and some may even threaten the parent by refusing them care, the ultimate choice still belongs to the parent. One of the most well-known alternative schedules you can follow was created by American pediatrician Dr. Robert Sears who wrote a book titled The Vaccine Book: Making the Right Decision for Your Child. In this book Dr. Sears lays out an alternative schedule that spreads out the shots for your child. The decision as to how to vaccinate (or if to) is a very important one to make and with as much education as possible.

Even with this small sampling of the vaccines on the childhood schedule it is clear that the risks versus benefits involved in making decisions for your children is not as clear cut as the vaccine apologists like to make it out for the typical person. If we only went by the information given to us through the media, internet or most pediatricians we would only see the benefits of the vaccines and we would never even look at the other side of this coin. Any information that goes contrary to the benefits is hidden deep or obfuscated so that what we perceive are only positives regarding the vaccines and this is a grave mis justice for all involved. The bottom line is that this is a subject well worth the time investment. Anyone who needs to make decisions regarding vaccines should have honest, balanced information that allows them to make an informed decision. When you are only given one side of an argument it makes it next to impossible to make the educated and accurate decisions that are necessary. The vaccine apologists do not want you to make informed decisions. What they want is for you to take their word that all is okay. They want you to simply trust them that they have you and your child's best interests at heart. You are certainly free to accept their word. Where you place blind trust is for the
individual to decide. For those who wish to look at evidence before making these important decisions, the information is there if you want it. You may have to look hard to find it but it is there for everyone who wishes to look for it. Happy hunting.

Point Number Sixteen
"You're not a real doctor."

"Blind obedience to authority is the greatest enemy of the truth," ~Albert Einstein, who also said, "It is the first responsibility of every citizen to question authority."

"Oh, you're a chiropractor. You're not a real doctor." If I had a dime for every time I heard that one. As a chiropractor, I have had to deal with this particular bias since graduating with my DOCTORATE (yes, I am a real doctor) in chiropractic over 25 years ago. For some, this is the only argument they can seem to come up with when they disagree with something I have stated. It is the "last ditch argument." I could attempt to explain that chiropractic schools have as many or more classroom hours as medical schools. I could try explaining that chiropractors have more training in many subjects and less in other subjects as medical doctors get in school. I could also try explaining that between education in school and additional training out of school, along with self study into topics, the need to have a specific degree is not always mandatory to having the requisite understanding of a particular topic. However, the individual who is making this kind of a statement rarely has any desire to hear this explanation and no desire to move past their particular bias.

This type of response is referred to as the credentials fallacy. "The credentials fallacy is a logical fallacy that occurs when someone dismisses an argument by stating that whoever made it doesn't have proper credentials, so their argument must be wrong or unimportant." This is very similar to "the appeal to authority, which occurs when an argument is claimed to necessarily be right, simply because it was made by someone who is perceived as an authority figure, and the appeal to accomplishments, which occurs when an arguement is claimed to necessarily be right, simply because it was made by someone with certain accomplishments (Example Dr. Fauci)." (1) There are many people who seem to think that being a medical doctor automatically gives you authority to speak on pretty much anything that is even remotely connected to health or sickness. This, of course, includes vaccines. Even many medical doctors seem to have this (high) opinion of themselves and their "right" to be authorities on subjects such as vaccines over any one else who does not have MD after their name. It is an interesting viewpoint since the standard of education for medical doctors when it comes to vaccines is so incredibly limited. It is also a viewpoint that was well and truly torn apart during covid (see Point Number Seventeen).

"According to a 2022 American Association of Medical Colleges Curriculum Inventory survey, 125 of 140 accredited medical institutions include some topics related to vaccines and immunization in their curriculum; however, there remains no standardized formal vaccine education in most medical programs." "This study was done at a large Pennsylvania medical school (School of Medicine, University of Pittsburgh) that, similar to most medical institutions, does not offer a formal vaccine curriculum in the preclinical or clinical years." "Many medical students reported insufficient knowledge of vaccine policy, vaccine development, and vaccine-focused initiatives at their school and within the community, with 40%–60% also reporting discomfort in discussing vaccines in clinical and nonclinical settings. Importantly, the need for further vaccine education was well recognized, with 79% reporting insufficient coverage of vaccine topics in the current curriculum." "Insufficient coverage of vaccines in medical school curricula has been reported in other institutions and countries. A total of 70% of German medical students reported dissatisfaction with teaching on vaccine hesitancy and communication strategies for vaccine information. A U.S. study found that only 40% of medical students expressed knowledge of the human papillomavirus vaccine, and 40% felt comfortable counseling patients. A survey of French medical students noted that one third felt unprepared to communicate with patients about vaccines or navigate vaccine hesitancy." (2) This certainly begins to place a different perspective on the notion of MD's being an authority on the subject of vaccines.

This viewpoint on the lack of vaccine education that MD's get while in school has been echoed by many medical doctors themselves. What follows are dozens of quotes from medical doctors, medical school instructors and others that fit the bill as "experts" on vaccines and what they have to say about their lack of education and training in the subject of vaccines and their own personal views against the vaccine program. Those who wish to continue placing medical doctors on the pedestal of vaccine authority should read through all of these quotes and then do a rethink on this erroneous belief:

"The only thing we learned in [medical] school was that there was a program and that we should follow that vaccine program. As to the vaccine itself and the contents of the vaccines, no we didn't study that. We assumed that what the pharmaceuticals (companies), that what they did and the CDC accepted, that that's the way it is."
~Ramon Ramos, MD and pediatric specialist. (3)

Paul Thomas, MD, author of several books on vaccines, recollected, "We got a lot of microbiology, we learned about diseases, and we learned that vaccines were the solution to those diseases that, what they say, are 'vaccine preventable.' But, actually, what was in the vaccines, I don't remember really learning anything. ... I was never taught, when I was in medical school 30 years ago, what was in a vaccine. We were only taught they're wonderful." (3)

"I can tell you, having been in a medical center, having taught biochemistry to medical students, and talking to hundreds of medical doctors, they get very little training in toxicology... I mean, no courses that are specifically designed, such as a PhD student in toxicology would have, or a PhD student in biochemistry. They don't understand it at all. They are not trained to evaluate the toxic effects of chemicals, especially at the research level. One, they don't do research programs, they don't have the insight that's developed and required for someone writing a PhD thesis in toxicology or biochemistry of materials that inhibit enzymes. They just don't understand the science and the chemistry at that level. And certainly pediatricians don't."
-biochemist Boyd Haley, PhD, who taught at the University of Kentucky Medical Center in Lexington (3)

"I don't remember them teaching me anything about adverse effects... at all," said Patricia Ryan, MD. "They just wanted you to memorize the schedule and make sure you knew when to give [the vaccines]." (3)

James Neuenschwander, MD recalled that, when he went to medical school more than 30 years ago, there was "not much training at all" on vaccines. "I don't know that it's changed very much, he said. "Basically, it was... here's the schedule. These are the saviors of mankind, they are safe, and you need to make sure everybody's vaccinated." (3)

"I never learned in medical school how vaccines were studied, what type of clinical trials they went through, how they evaluated adverse reactions... how they even evaluated effectiveness. So, after Victoria (her daughter) died, I started reading everything that is put out there. Anything that would lead me to a topic, then I would Google that topic... and if there were textbooks in relation to that topic, I would order them and then, based on reading that book, I would order another book. What I have learned has shocked me." -Stephanie Christner, DO, whose infant daughter did not survive vaccination (3)

"We were told that vaccines are safe and effective, here's the schedule, ignore the inserts... that's lawyer jargon," recalled Cammy Benton, MD. "I think in medical school you're learning so much that it's kind of difficult to learn, that you assumed [with] vaccines the science was settled, tried and true. So you just didn't question it, that was the easy part... okay, this is for sure. So you just accept it." "We learned what [vaccines] were, what the diseases were," said Joseph Mercola, DO. "We probably learned more about the diseases and, of course, everyone accepted the dogma that vaccines work. There was just no critical analysis about the pros and cons. It was never discussed, let alone the side effects." (3)

"I decided to go to the CDC, and discovered that most of what I'd accepted as the truth about vaccines really wasn't true at all: that vaccines weren't responsible for the eradication of polio and smallpox, and haven't been proven safe; that vaccines deemed "effective" may still not protect against the disease; that research studies use a second vaccine as placebo, not an inert substance; and that vaccines are not harmless, that many thousands have been injured and many hundreds have died as a result of them." – Sherri Tenpenny, DO, Saying No to Vaccines, 2008, "A Note to Readers."

"You'd be amazed at the number of physicians, you ask them what's in a vaccine?" said neurosurgeon Russell Blaylock, MD. " They'll say, well, there's the bacteria, the virus you want to vaccinate against, and then there's a little immune stimulant in there to help stimulate the immunity so they react against those viral antigens." "They don't know about these other chemicals in there like formaldehyde, special proteins, special lipids that are known to be brain toxic, that are known to induce autoimmunity in the brain. They're not aware of that. They don't know that MSG is in a lot of vaccines—monosodium glutamate, a brain excitotoxin. They're not aware of what's in the vaccine they're giving." (4)

"There is no convincing scientific evidence that mass inoculation can be credited with eliminating any childhood disease. It's true that some diseases have diminished or disappeared in the US since inoculations were introduced, but one must ask why they did so simultaneously in Europe, where mass immunization did not take place. There are significant risks associated with every immunization. Yet doctors administer them routinely without warning parents or determining whether they're contraindicated for that particular child. No one knows the long-term consequence of injecting foreign proteins into the body of your child, and no one is making any structured effort to find out. There is growing suspicion that immunization against relatively harmless childhood diseases may be responsible for the dramatic increase in autoimmune diseases, cancer, leukemia, rheumatoid arthritis, Lou Gehrig's Disease, lupus, and Guillain-Barre syndrome. Have we traded mumps and measles for cancer and leukemia?"

~From Dr. R. Mendelsohn, MD (pediatrician) book *How to Raise a Healthy Child … in Spite of Your Doctor*, 1984.

"The most memorable event was in the winter of 2009, when the H1N1 flu vaccine was given. Three patients in close succession were wheeled into the ER with total kidney shutdown. When I talked to them, each one volunteered, "I was fine until I had that vaccine." All three had shown normal kidney function in their outpatient records, and all three required dialysis. Two recovered, and one died of complications several months later. I began taking vaccine histories on all my patients, and was often startled by what I heard. Several had been admitted with normal kidneys but had their health decline within 24 hours of the vaccine, and even these well-defined and documented cases were denied as vaccine-induced by my colleagues, except for the rare doctor or nurse who would agree with me in private, when nobody was listening. I resolved to find out everything I could about safety trials for vaccines. What I learned led me to leave my practice and become a full-time researcher on vaccination and the immune system." – from *Dissolving Illusions – Disease, Vaccines, and the Forgotten History,* Dr. Suzanne Humphries, MD & Roman Bystrianyk (Introduction, pp. xii-xiv).

"I used to tell them that there were, indeed, adverse reactions, associated with the vaccine – I was not one of those doctors who would gloss over such unpleasant details – but that we doctors were told that the adverse reactions that might occur after the pertussis vaccine were at least ten times less likely than the chance of getting complications from having the disease, and that, essentially, the point of giving their child the vaccine was to prevent them from getting the disease. Indeed, I used to think that parents who didn't want to vaccinate their children were either ignorant, or sociopathic. I believe that view is not uncommon among doctors today. Why did I have this attitude? Well, throughout my medical training I was taught that the people who used to die in their thousands or hundreds of thousands from diseases like diphtheria, whooping cough and measles – diseases for which there are vaccines – stopped dying because of the introduction of vaccines."

~Dr. Jayne L.M. Donegan in her foreword to the book *Dissolving Illusions – Disease, Vaccines, and the Forgotten History*

"Children seen in the vaccine clinic would come to our ER with seizures, respiratory arrest, and asthma attacks. I began to realize that not all children respond well to vaccines, and that some die. Later I began to see the fraud and corruption in the Advisory Committees and in how vaccines are marketed. I had no idea that those killed and injured had no recourse against either manufacturer or physician. Manufacturers enjoy full immunity from lawsuits, and the Vaccine Court is almost a secret, yet has paid out $3 billion since 1986. [Now over $4 B.] The VAERS system is also poorly advertised and the government admits it receives only about 10% of the adverse events that occur. We mandate more vaccines than any other country, and have a higher infant mortality rate than some third world countries. Most kids do OK, but some don't. Genetics and timing are also important; no drug or dosage is right for everyone. Federal cases against drug companies show that safety data are hidden, manipulated, and even fabricated. Most safety studies use fake placebos, like aluminum adjuvant for HPV, or a Meningitis Vaccine for Pneumo. All independent meta-analyses say that real safety studies are needed. There are 200+ new vaccines in the pipeline, and all of them will be approved, recommended, and mandated. Isn't enough enough?" ~from Dr. Toni Bark, MD, Letter to Oregon State Senator Ferrioli, posted in Health Impact News Oct. 22, 2015.

"I was taught that vaccines were completely safe and effective, and for years I used them. But my experience and what parents and doctors were telling me, was that vaccines aren't completely safe or effective. We were taught that polio, smallpox, and most infectious diseases went away because of vaccines. But the literature shows that diphtheria, tetanus, polio, pertussis, measles, influenza, TB, and scarlet fever were already waning before antibiotics and vaccines, because of clean water, better living conditions, sanitation, and nutrition. Other studies show that antibodies aren't how the body is protected, and that some vaccines contain foreign DNA that accumulates in the body and brain, and impairs the immune system. What we have now is a one-sided way of thinking that doesn't allow debate. It's heartbreaking to see kids who were speaking, doing well, and developmentally normal, who lost their voice, made no eye contact, developed seizures, asthma, and allergies, and had nowhere to go because the doctor said it was a coincidence. The studies that deny any correlation between vaccination and autism don't meet scientific standards." ~Lawrence B. Palevsky, M.D., pediatrician.

"I could go on and on; ... The roster of family doctors, pediatricians, and other doctors speaking out against mandatory vaccinations and questioning the official dogma surrounding them grows larger by the day. No matter where and in what matter they practice, or what their specialty, their arguments and objections are all remarkably similar, invoking and elaborating on the very same themes that Dr. Mendelsohn, presciently identified a generation ago. Rather than opposing all vaccines across the board, they favor a pro-choice position, as I do: they want safer vaccines, expose cover-ups, demand full disclosure by the industry and the CDC, insist on informed consent, and oppose making vaccination mandatory. And hiding behind them stand many more who feel the same way but are afraid to say so openly. In one study that interviewed general pediatricians and pediatric subspecialists, 10% of the former and 21% of the latter admitted that they would not follow the CDC mandates in vaccinating their own children in the future; many planned to postpone the MMR at least until after 18 months of age, and to reject the rotavirus, meningococcus, and hepatitis A vaccines altogether." (The stats are from Martin, M. and Badalyan, V. in "Vaccination Practices Among Physicians and Their Children," *Open Journal of Pediatrics* 2:228, 2012.) ~Dr. Richard Moskowitz, MD and author of multiple books.

"As you know, medical doctors don't have a lot training in vaccines. We don't have a lot of training in anything in detail unless you become a specialist. I've been reading about vaccines since 2009, about an hour a day. I started reading about vaccines when I saw my patients getting hurt, and that was really hard for me. I didn't want to believe it. ... In the [...] two years [after I began my practice], I noticed that there was a separation in my patient population. There were patients who were seeing the local chiropractor who were healthier than my other patients, and they were doing some other things for their health other than just taking medication for whatever condition they might have. They also had a lower vaccine uptake and they were healthy. And that was really hard for me to recognize." -Dr. Robert Zajac, MD is a U.S. pediatrician.

"With what I now know, I cannot support mandatory vaccines for children. Some kids respond well to vaccines, but others do not. How can we be sure who will and who will not? Should we really sacrifice one for many? Parents have to have the right to choose! Parents have to make their own informed decisions. Parents deserve access to this information which has been buried so deep that even I, a practicing physician, hadn't been aware of." "People keep asking me if I'm scared to speak about this. My realest fear is that we will continue to assume that these moms are making this stuff up."
~Dr. Rachel Ross, MD & PhD, taken from the movie Vaxxed.

"I never imagined myself in this position, least so in the very beginning of my Ph.D. research training in immunology. In fact, at that time, I was very enthusiastic about the concept of vaccination, just like any typical immunologist. However, after years of doing research in immunology, observing scientific activities of my superiors, and analyzing vaccine issues, I realized that vaccination is one of the most deceptive inventions that science could ever convince the world to accept." ~Dr. Tetyana Obukhanych, Ph.D.in epidemiology and author of *Vaccine Illusion.* (5)

"There are absolutely no good vaccines anywhere. They are dangerous for health. There is no science behind vaccines. They cause the diseases they are supposed to prevent, plus a host of other diseases, like AIDS. No vaccines are necessary, all vaccines are a hoax. " ~Dr. Shiv Chopra, PhD microbiologist, former vaccine researcher for Health Canada (the Canadian FDA) , WHO fellow, former vaccine maker, whistle blower and author of '*CORRUPT TO THE CORE: Memoirs of a Health Canada Whistleblower.*' (5)

In February of 2025, Dr. Alvin Moss, MD, a professor at the West Virginia University (WVU) School of Medicine, testified in front of West Virginia lawmakers against legislation to remove all religious and philosophical exemptions for vaccination. He argued that the medical community ignores scientific research about vaccine injuries, stating "They know the vaccines come with serious adverse events, they've seen them in their children." (6) Dr. Moss also wrote an excellent article titled 20 Problems with Vaccination which details his understanding of vaccine risks. (7)

"You should be FIGHTING LIKE HELL for the safety of our children from even the most remote possibility that vaccines aren't as safe as they could be or aren't as safe as we are being told. Instead of fighting for truth and safety, you're fighting like rats for your piece of cheese." ~Jim Meehan, MD, taken from his message to all pediatricians.(8)

"Time to wake up and smell the coffee. The largest contributor to SIDS is vaccines and if you can't see that you are blind. The vast majority of SIDS ~ 80% occur within a week of a vaccine." ~Dr. James Thorp, MD (from his X page)

"Every day I speak to parents whose children were destroyed by vaccines. Heed my warnings." ~Dr. Andrew Zywiec, M.D. (from his X page)

"For decades, VAERS has underreported vaccine injuries—yet Pharma & hospital systems tried to silence doctors who exposed it." ~Dr. Simone Gold, MD (from her X page)

"I will never believe it's okay for the government to decide what goes into your body." ~Dr. Joseph Ladapo, MD, Florida's Surgeon General, (from his X page)

"There's a deep sadness in watching the righteous fervor of doctors and pharmacists—unwitting victims of decades of Pharma disinformation—directed not at who deceived them, but at newly informed, so-called "misinformationists" who recovered from it, are now immune, and tell truths" "For over a century, they've known vaccines suddenly kill infants. Since then, health officials have done all they can to cover it up and gaslight the parents." ~Dr. Pierre Kory, MD (from his X page)

"LOUDER! MANDATES are NOT HEALTHCARE!" ~Dr. Mollie James, MD (from her X page)

"...unvaccinated children are far healthier than those who are vaccinated." ~Kelly Victory, MD (from her X page)

"I don't do Halloween, but if I did I would be a vaccine insert…those things are pretty scary." ~Dr. Jeff Barke, MD. (from his Instagram)

'Personally, I will never get another vaccine again." ~Dr. Mary Talley Bowden, MD (from her X page)

This list is only a small fraction of the trained professionals, MD's, PhD. 's, who have spoken out against the dangers, mandates and censorship that surround the vaccine program. None of these individuals woke up one morning and said, "hey, I think I will ruin my career and possibly my entire life today." Many of these individuals have been fired from their positions and/or essentially blackballed from the medical and scientific community for having the courage to speak out. All of these individuals were respected in their communities right up to the second before they spoke out and then suddenly, overnight, they were deemed "quacks," frauds, charlatans and "anti-vaxxers."

Lastly, I want to highlight two of these individuals who have risked their careers, their lively-hoods, to speak out about the dangers of vaccines. I am highlighting these two specifically because of their incredible backgrounds, the respect they had earned in their communities prior to speaking out and their notoriety currently. Both of these individuals have had stellar careers and try and try as hard as the media and others try to discredit them (and they are); they still can not erase their spectacular backgrounds.

Dr. Peter McCullough is an internist, cardiologist, epidemiologist holding degrees from Baylor University, University of Texas Southwestern Medical School, University of Michigan, and Southern Methodist University. In 2014, Dr. McCullough joined Baylor Scott & White Health as Vice Chief of Internal Medicine at BUMC, Chief of Cardiovascular Research of the Baylor Heart and Vascular Institute, and Program Director of the cardiovascular disease fellowship program at BUMC (he was released from contract when he began speaking out about the covid vaccines). Dr. McCullough is recognized internationally as a leading figure in the study of chronic kidney disease as a cardiovascular risk state, having over 1,000 publications to his name and over 500 citations in the National Library of Medicine. He is also a founder of the Cardio Renal Society of America, which is a group that dedicates itself to bringing cardiologists and nephrologists together to work on the increasing global issue of cardiorenal syndromes. He was the Co-Editor of Reviews in Cardiovascular Medicine and is also currently serving as the Chair of the National Kidney Foundation's Kidney Early Evaluation Program (KEEP), the largest community screening effort for chronic diseases in America. (9)

Dr. McCullough has been all over the news since the pandemic and has testified multiple times in the US Senate, US House of Representatives and multiple state assemblies on the dangers of the covid vaccines. He has also been one of the most prolific researchers in regards to these dangers as well. Meanwhile, the mainstream media largely presents a negative view of him as a conspiracy theorist and a spreader of misinformation.

Dr. Robert Malone, M.D., Pathology; M.S., Virology, Immunology, Molecular Biology, is the discoverer of in-vitro and in-vivo RNA transfection and the inventor of mRNA vaccines, while he was at the Salk Institute in 1988. His research was continued at Vical in 1989, where the first in-vivo mammalian experiments were designed by him. The mRNA, constructs, reagents were developed at the Salk institute and Vical by Dr. Malone. The initial patent disclosures were written by Dr. Malone in 1988-1989. Dr. Malone was also an inventor of DNA vaccines in 1988 and 1989. This work has resulted in over 10 patents and numerous publications, yielding about 7,000 citations. He received his medical training at Northwestern University (M.D.) and Harvard University (Clinical Research Post Graduate) medical school, and in pathology at the University of California at Davis. Davis. Dr. Malone is currently one of the Committee members for the Advisory Committee on Immunization Practices(ACIP), a committee of experts that provides vaccine and immunization recommendations to the CDC and Department of Health and Human Services (HHS). The media's view of him can be summed up perfectly with this quote from Politi-fact, "Malone's rise to right-wing stardom and subsequent fall into social media purgatory underscore how accomplished doctors can exploit their credentials to spread harmful misinformation."

Dr. McCullough and Dr. Malone (as well as many others) are both perfect examples of what has been referred to as "being Wakefielded." This, of course, is in reference to the actions that were taken against Dr. Andrew Wakefield (Point 11). No matter how stellar a person's career, if they raise a question that goes against the vaccine agenda they will be set upon and their future forever altered. Yet these individuals have all chosen to speak up regardless of the consequences and risks to their lives and livelihoods. This takes more courage and makes their words even more powerful than any of the pharma schills who continue to speak ill words against those that go against the vaccine orthodoxy. It truly is the perfect example of how this topic of vaccines can not be discussed with any real rationality. It is probably the only topic in science that if you disagree with the talking points, you can not be a part of the conversation at all. If you were to look back at the history of any of the people listed in this chapter you could doubtless find multiple examples of subjects (other than vaccines) that any of these individuals may have spoken up about throughout the course of their careers. You would then find that other than some minor debating of points or other minor and meaningless contention over these points, nothing happened to them of their careers or reputations. However, go against the vaccine orthodoxy, speak out even once against vaccines, and all hell breaks loose. You really want to go down the whole "you're not a real doctor" path? The phrase is meaningless in light of all of those that "fit your bill" who are speaking up and speaking out against this orthodoxy.

Point Number Seventeen
The SARs-CoV-2 Agenda

F.E.A.R.
False Evidence Appearing Real

I thought it fitting to end with a Point regarding these last few years that the world has experienced during SARs-CoV-2. For me, and for so many others in the Health Freedom movement, these last few years have felt like the culmination of decades of activity (and not in a good way). I actually had to put down the writing of this book during 2020 because I was becoming too incensed with everything that was going on and the act of writing this book was keeping me too closely attached to the situation. Even though it was next to impossible to completely detach from what was going on, the book was just too much for me at the time. I took a full two years off from writing before I felt the urge to finish what I had started. I am sure most people would not have understood why I was affected by everything as I was, but perhaps once you have absorbed all of the material from this book you may be able to see how this current environment was the sour frosting on top of the proverbial cake for those who had already been immersed in all of this information prior to the events in question.

As I mentioned way back in Point 1, beginning from 2015 there was a very strong push within the government to enact legislation to enforce the vaccine mandates. States were actively working to not only take away the exemptions but they were also pursuing other legislation to make it easier to get the vaccines into children without the consent of parents. (1, 2) At the same time the government was trying to tighten their grip regarding exemptions, they were also attacking homeschooling. (3, 4, 5) This was simply another avenue into regulating how children could get vaccinated. Many parents who choose to homeschool do this for a variety of reasons, religion being one of the top reasons, however a large percentage of homeschoolers do choose to not vaccinate their children and this was entirely unacceptable by those in charge. From the early 2000s right up until the end of 2019, the percentage of people not getting vaccinated did not change much at all (6), however what did change was the response from those who did not want their medical freedoms taken away. The amount of protests and activism increased to the point that the World Health Organization (WHO) actually named vaccine hesitancy to their top ten global threats for the year 2019. (7) Yes, the 1-2% of people who were unvaccinated ranked as being a "global threat" equal to global warming. The real issue for them was that the message regarding the potential dangers of vaccines was beginning to get out to mainstream America and the pharmaceutical companies and the government did not like what was happening one little bit.

Enter 2020. The first confirmed case of SARs-CoV-2 in the U.S. was on January 21, 2020, however we now know that there were cases as early as December 2019. By March 11 the WHO had declared a pandemic and by March 13 a state of national emergency was declared for the U.S.(8) From here things seemed to escalate exponentially, and as things escalated, anything that was said that went against the narrative being created by the government led to intense criticism and retaliation. The following quote underscores this reality, "The White House is asking social media companies to clamp down on chatter that deviates from officially distributed COVID-19 information as part of President Biden's "wartime effort" to vanquish the coronavirus. A senior administration official tells Reuters that the Biden administration is asking Facebook, Twitter and Google to help prevent anti-vaccine fears from going viral, as distrust of the inoculations emerges as a major barrier in the fight against the deadly virus."(9) Even the executive editor of the prestigious British Medical Journal (BMJ) was troubled by what was happening, "Science is being suppressed for political and financial gain. Covid-19 has unleashed state corruption on a grand scale, and it is harmful to public health. Politicians and industry are responsible for this opportunistic embezzlement. So too are scientists and health experts. The pandemic has revealed how the medical-political complex can be manipulated in an emergency—a time when it is even more important to safeguard science." (10) There was even an interesting study that came out of New Zealand around this time that looked at people's reactions to information they felt supported government efforts to eliminate SARs-CoV-2 versus information that challenged these ideas. Even when presented with information that was essentially equal and valid and the only difference being which perspective was being presented, the reactions from individuals being assessed showed that "these effects were mediated by moral outrage, supporting that elimination efforts have become moralized." (11) This study illustrated how the simple idea of questioning the narrative had become "moralized." It really helps to explain the reactions of so many people to the questioning of the information that was being disseminated at this time. What I would like to do here is break down some of the finer points around the virus and the restrictions and attempt to illustrate how well this entire situation has shown how the government and the pharmaceutical companies act in concert with each other in regard to viruses and vaccines. With the media and the government screaming beware of the conspiracy theorists, the events around SARs-CoV-2 were a perfect example of everything I have written about up to here. So here's a list of some of the things that were being labeled as conspiracy and "fake news" on the various media platforms. Any of these topics could have potentially had you removed from the various media platforms and/or ostracized by your friends or society . Wearing masks. Vaccine safety or efficacy. The virus leaked from a lab. Natural immunity. Boosters. Covid deaths. Ivermectin and hydroxychloroquine. Dr. Fauci waffling on recommendations. If anything you said on these topics did not conform to the party line, you were at risk of being banished from social media, losing your job and of ridicule from those around you for being a conspiracy nut job. So let's do the deep dive into some of these "conspiracy" ideas and see how well that moniker holds up under actual scrutiny.

Conspiracy idea #1 SARs-CoV-2 is a virus of the elderly and infirmed
Conspiracy idea #2 SARs-CoV-2 deaths are inflated numbers

As these two statements tend to go along with each other I will address them together. One of the first things that is necessary to understand when looking at SARs-CoV-2 is the difference between case fatality rate (CFR) and incidence fatality rate (IFR). CFR is based on the confirmed deaths among the confirmed cases of a specific disease, whereas IFR is the number of confirmed deaths out of all of the people possibly infected with the disease. Although IFR is often harder to establish since you need to estimate asymptomatic and undiagnosed persons as well as confirmed cases, it creates a far more realistic understanding of the virulence of a disease than the CFR does. During the first few months of SARs-CoV-2 the media repeatedly stated that the death rate from Covid-19 was around 2-4% (12,13) Unfortunately, most Americans probably did not understand the difference between what was being given (CFR) and what was not being given at the time (IFR). This reporting of high CFR numbers to the public created unnecessary anxiety, especially as it was typically not explained from the perspective of CFR vs IFR. The current information now shows that SARs-CoV-2, globally has an IFR somewhere between 0.03-0.07%.(14) This is almost exactly the IFR for the seasonal flu. (15) That is a far cry from the 2-4% that was being thrown around at the beginning of the pandemic.

Another factor that needs to be considered when looking at the deaths from Covid-19 is who is being affected by the virus. It became apparent rather quickly that this virus is a very selective bug and not everyone was being affected in the same manner. Not only was an individual's age a major player but their overall health was a huge factor as well. "CDC Director Rochelle Walensky admitted that over 75% of "COVID deaths" occurred in people "who had at least four comorbidities. So really, these are people who are unwell to begin with," she stated. (16) This was information that was known as early as June of 2020 as seen in this quote from a journal paper which noted "that persons with underlying chronic illnesses are more likely to contract the virus and become severely ill." (17) Or this one from July 2020 from the *Journal of Aging Clinical and Experimental Research* which states that, "the high mortality rate of COVID-19 among the elderly, we believe that it may be related to the high prevalence of comorbidities among the elderly." (18) And my favorite quote regarding age and health status which clearly stated that "higher COVID-19 mortality among older adults was partially explained by other risk factors. 'Healthy' older adults were at much lower risk. Nonetheless, older age was an independent risk factor for COVID-19 mortality." (19)

The simple fact is that complications and death from SARs-CoV-2 almost exclusively affects older individuals with preexisting health conditions. The Mayo Clinic stated that "in the U.S. about 81% of deaths from the disease have been in people aged 65 and older, and that risks are even higher for older people when they have other health conditions." (20) Worldwide only 1% of deaths from Covid-19 occurred in the group of individuals aged between 15-44. (21) Even the CDC, BMJ and JAMA understand that this is a virus that by and large affects the sick and elderly. (22,23,24) Does this mean that no one who was seemingly healthy or was under the age of 55 died from Covid-19? Of course not, in all diseases there are always what are referred to as outliers. Outliers are those who are severely affected by a virus who are outside of the normally expected patterns of involvement. This is a completely expected circumstance with any virus. The issue is not whether you can die from SARs-CoV-2 but rather what are your true risks of dying from Covid-19. "For COVID-19, outliers are relatively rare—for example, out of more than 11,800 deaths reported in New York City by late April (2020), only 10 were under age 44 and had no underlying condition." (25) It is this knowledge that should have been informing not only governmental policy, but the public's reactions as well. Those who were at extreme risk of dying from SARs-CoV-2 should have been the focus and concern not locking down society and creating panic among those whose risks were negligible. The ripple effects of the fear created during the pandemic are still being felt and will most likely continue to be felt for many years to come.

The last part regarding deaths is the inflation of the totals. Putting this information together with the previous information really allows you to look at the deadliness of SARs-CoV-2 with new eyes. I do not think anyone will argue that far too many people have died from Covid-19 and that each and everyone of these deaths is a tragedy. The world wide death totals are staggering. But are the death toll numbers being presented accurate or are they inaccurate. This is the real question and it is an important one when looking at the virus's virulence. When it comes to questioning the accuracy of the death totals, you can find plenty of stories to make you question things. An article in the Washington Examiner had this to say regarding inflated numbers, "Two Minnesota state lawmakers are calling for an audit of death certificates that were attributed to the coronavirus, saying COVID-19 deaths could have been inflated by 40%. State Rep. Mary Franson and state Sen. Scott Jensen released a video last week revealing that after reviewing thousands of death certificates in the state, 40% did not have COVID-19 as the underlying cause of death." (26) A similar article in the *Washington Post* shared information about other states with questionable records, "In Alabama, officials have ruled that one of every 10 people who died with covid-19 did not die of covid-19. Colorado, by contrast, has included some deaths where the disease caused by the novel coronavirus was deemed probable — based on symptoms and possible exposure — but not confirmed through a test. Ohio, Connecticut and Delaware have since begun reporting deaths of people who were presumed infected but had not been tested." (27) Adding to this is an article from the *Los Angeles Times* which had this to say on the subject, "Los Angeles County public health officials said their tally of COVID-19 deaths includes any person who died from a heart attack, stroke or another ailment if they had tested positive for the coronavirus within the last 90 days. In Oregon, state public health officials said they include anyone who had tested positive within 60 days of death, including those who died from accidents such as automobile wrecks. Already there is evidence that it isn't just the virus — attributed to more than 200,000 deaths in the numbers reported by states so far — that has ended American lives too soon." (28) To make matters worse Dr. Deborah Birx, who was the White House Coronavirus Response Coordinator under President Donald Trump, actually said this at a press conference, "the intent is right now that if someone dies with COVID-19 we are counting that as a COVID-19 death." (29) Notice that she says "with" Covid-19, not "from" Covid-19. The last piece of this puzzle comes straight from the CDC themselves as per the instructions that were sent out to all hospitals and doctors in regard to how to fill out death certificates during Covid. "Part I and II of a death certificate ask what caused a death and what other factors contributed to it. If COVID-19 appears among the causes and contributors, CDC guidance counts that as a COVID-19-related death." (30) To go along with this information regarding the death certificates, there was even the question whether hospitals were actually making money off of Covid deaths. *USA Today* did one of their Fact Checks and reported that, "We rate the claim that hospitals get paid more if patients are listed as COVID-19 and on ventilators as TRUE. Hospitals and doctors do get paid more for Medicare patients diagnosed with COVID-19 or if it's considered presumed, they have COVID-19 absent a laboratory-confirmed test, and three times more if the patients are placed on a ventilator to cover the cost of care and loss of business resulting from a shift in focus to treat COVID-19 cases." (31) This piece of information adds an entirely new dimension to this issue and makes you wonder how much motivation hospitals had to label something as a death from Covid.

The bottom line here is that the current IFR for SARs-CoV-2 is being reported as between 0.03-0.07%, which is incredibly low. This IFR is reached by using the current death toll numbers that are clearly questionable. This leads one to assume that the IFR would be even lower if the data was more accurate. Assuming this to be true this makes the actual virulence of SARs-CoV-2 even less than is being reported. Can SARs-CoV-2 kill someone, yes. Has it killed far too many people, yes. But the issue here is that the actual risks of being killed from this virus are far lower than it is being made to look like to the public. This is especially true for those that are healthy and under the age of 55. For people in this category the risks for SARs-CoV-2 are incredibly low. If we look at children with this virus we see that it is less dangerous for them than the seasonal flu can be, yet the push for shutting down schools and now for making the Covid vaccines part

Covid vaccines part of the mandatory schedule is huge. Ask yourself why that is?

Conspiracy idea #3 Masks are not an effective protection for SARs-CoV-2
Conspiracy idea #4 Six feet distancing is a joke

This one really got a lot of airplay early on and was one of the more contentious issues that was brought up during all of the mandates. Wearing a mask became a kind of badge of honor among some people. If you were against wearing masks you were seen as being against saving lives. The big question here however is do (did) the masks actually save lives. I am putting the "six foot rule" in with the masks since it was another safety rule that seemed to be plucked from the air and had as much to do with keeping us safe as did wearing a bandana wrapped around your face.

Early on in the pandemic many people in our government did not recommend the wearing of masks. In fact the Surgeon General, Jerome Adams, even went as far as saying masks were "NOT effective in preventing [the] general public from catching Coronavirus." (32) Even Dr. Fauci himself stated that, "when you're in the middle of an outbreak, wearing a mask might make people feel a little bit better and it might even block a droplet, but it's not providing the perfect protection that people think that it is." (33) It was in fact, Dr. Fauci who did an about-face and not only decided people should wear masks but also began moralizing them. Fauci was quoted as saying, "I want to protect myself and protect others, and also because I want to make it be a symbol for people to see that that's the kind of thing you should be doing," he also stated that those who were not wearing a mask "increases the risk of there being transmissibility." (34, 35) These comments were less than a month after his first comments regarding not wearing a mask. I often wondered what revelatory piece of research occurred during that time period that so altered his view point. Even the World Health Organization (WHO) was initially against the wearing of masks, "There is no specific evidence to suggest that the wearing of masks by the mass population has any potential benefit. In fact, there's some evidence to suggest the opposite in the misuse of wearing a mask properly or fitting it properly," Dr. Mike Ryan, executive director of the WHO health emergencies program, said at a media briefing in Geneva, Switzerland." (36) Europe's version of the CDC had this to say in regards to wearing masks, "There is limited evidence on the effectiveness of medical face masks for the prevention of COVID-19 in the community." (37) Even some of the media was hip to what the research was saying about masks at the time, "While the science behind whether masks can prevent a person from catching the coronavirus hasn't changed (a mask does not help a healthy person avoid infection), public guidance may be shifting." (38) The fact is that prior to this pandemic there was a total consensus in the scientific literature regarding the lack of effectiveness of the public wearing face masks. (39, 40, 41, 42, 43) Even after the pandemic began the science was still illustrating the ineffectiveness of wearing masks to stop the spread of viruses. (44, 45, 46, 47, 48, 49, 50, 51)

So did the science change? Was there some sudden 180 when it came to the effectiveness of wearing masks to stop the spread of the virus? The simple answer is no. This quote from an article in the *New England Journal of Medicine* seemed to sum things up pretty well, "It is also clear that masks serve symbolic roles. Masks are not only tools, they are also talismans that may help increase health care workers' perceived sense of safety, well-being, and trust in their hospitals. Although such reactions may not be strictly logical, we are all subject to fear and anxiety, especially during times of crisis. One might argue that fear and anxiety are better countered with data and education than with a marginally beneficial mask, particularly in light of the worldwide mask shortage, but it is difficult to get clinicians to hear this message in the heat of the current crisis." (52) Wearing masks was something that allowed the government to show they were doing something. Unfortunately the only thing it was actually providing was a false sense of security and a deep rooted sense of fear. As for masks saving lives, a study by the CDC actually showed that "85% of those who were confirmed as Covid-19 positive cases wore masks either"often "or" always." (53)

There are also risks to wearing the masks that should have been considered. You would have then been able to do a risk to benefit assessment to see if it is really worth wearing a mask and especially if it is worth mandating that everyone wears a mask. The World Health Organization came out with a list of "potential disadvantages" to wearing a mask that included "headache and/or breathing difficulties, development of facial skin lesions, irritant dermatitis or worsening acne, a false sense of security leading to potentially lower adherence to other critical preventive measures, disadvantages for those with mental illness, persons with cognitive impairment, those with asthma or chronic respiratory or breathing problems." (54) A German study found "severe psychological damage" in regard to mandatory mask usage. (55) An Italian study found higher than acceptable levels of inhaled CO2 from using masks. (56) And another German study found that the reusing of masks increased the risks of "self-contamination." (57) And you know darn well that everyone was reusing their masks. With all of the potential risks to wearing a mask combined with not only the very low protective value of wearing a mask, but also the very low virulence of the virus itself, makes it hard to understand the logic behind forcing people to wear them, especially children., which this more recent study points out with its conclusion, "child mask mandates fail a basic risk-benefit analysis. Recommending child masking to prevent the spread of COVID-19 is unsupported by current scientific data and inconsistent with accepted ethical norms." (58)

As for the six foot distance rule, just as with the studies regarding the lack of effectiveness of masks, studies regarding the spray of aerosols prior to and during the pandemic showed that this rule of six feet was at best arbitrary and at worse totally useless. "Sophisticated imaging studies have shown that plumes of aerosols are generated by sneezing or coughing. The aerosol plume contains the highest concentration of particles, which then dissipate in the air over time and distance. That distance is now much farther than previously appreciated, traveling up to 7–8 m (21-24 feet). A re-analysis of the size of particles emitted by an average person that would fall to the ground within 2 m is 60–100 µm, and these can be carried more than 6 m (18 feet) away by sneezing." (59) Notice that the distancesthat are mentioned in this particular research paper are between 18-24 feet. We are talking distances that are up to four times further than the mandated six feet rule we were told would protect us from exposure. The research evidence has been clear for many years that aerosols from coughs and sneezes can travel much further than the six feet of protection claimed by the government. (59, 60, 61) As with the mandating of masks, the rule of six feet was an attempt to do something, anything, in the face of a potentially deadly virus. Unfortunately, both of these measures did not respect the science that showed these measures to be weak answers to the problem. While the measures did next to nothing to curb the transmission of the virus they did irreversible damage to the psyche of the public. Children were especially vulnerable to this damage. Increases in anxiety, depression and suicide are just some of the damaging outcomes from the mandates and the fear during the pandemic. (62, 63, 64, 65, 66) Only time will tell us what the long term damage that has been done by initiating these procedures that have no clear scientific support simply for the act of "doing something."

Conspiracy idea #5 SARs-CoV-2 was released from a lab in China

When I first heard someone suggest that the virus had been created in a lab and then released, I had two initial reactions. My first reaction was to say that there was no way someone, especially our government, would do something like this on purpose. My second reaction was to think that I would not put it past our government to do anything to have their agenda reached. Now this does not mean that this is what happened. I will say at the time of this writing we do not know beyond any doubt exactly where the virus came from or if there was any sinister intent behind it. However, when people first began talking about the possibility that the virus was created and released (accident or on purpose) from the Wuhan Institute of Virology (WIV) in Wuhan, China, the instantaneous response from the politicians and the media was to deny and shame anyone who mentioned this crazy idea. Senator Tom Cotton was probably the very first person who was brave enough to openly discuss hypotheses regarding where the virus came from. Even though Sen. Cotton was only speaking openly about possible origins of Covid he was labeled a conspiracy theorist and called out in the media. (67) Another of the first individuals to speak out openly about the virus being of lab origin was James Lyons-Weiler, PhD who in February of 2020 published evidence of a genomic sequence pointing to a lab origin. (68) His information was immediately set upon by a team of scientists from China. (69) Even (then) President Trump was criticized for speaking publicly on this topic. This was all the press needed to further deride this as a conspiracy theory. When such a concentrated effort is being made to silence and discredit individuals who are making what certainly seemed at the time to be a reasonable hypothesis, you have to have at least a bit of suspicion as to their motivations. At the beginning of any type of investigation the first thing you do is to hash out any reasonable hypothesis and the only reason to immediately shut down someone who is trying to hash out a reasonable hypothesis is if they are trying to hide something.

Being referred to as a "crazy conspiracist" for even suggesting that the virus was anything but a natural occurrence was certainly not what I was after, so even though I talked non-stop about all of the other points I mention here, I kept my mouth shut about this particular point. Since the actual proof at the beginning of the pandemic was sparse, I wanted to see how this theory was going to play out before speaking out with an opinion. So where does this theory stand at the writing of this book? Here is what a recent headline in the *Wall Street Journal (WSJ)* said, "Lab Leak Most Likely Origin of Covid-19 Pandemic, Energy Department Now Says." According to the *WSJ*, "The U.S. Energy Department has concluded that the Covid pandemic most likely arose from a laboratory leak, according to a classified intelligence report recently provided to the White House and key members of Congress." They go on to add that, "The Energy Department's conclusion is the result of new intelligence and is significant because the agency has considerable scientific expertise and oversees a network of U.S. national laboratories, some of which conduct advanced biological research." (70) To add to this new revelation the *WSJ* also wrote another article titled, "FBI Director Says Covid Pandemic Likely Caused by Chinese Lab Leak." This article goes on to quote the FBI director as saying, "The FBI has for quite some time now assessed that the origins of the pandemic are most likely a potential lab incident in Wuhan." (71) While this new information may not conclusively prove that the virus came from the lab in Wuhan, it certainly should make everyone who thought it was a crazy conspiracy idea rethink their comments. It should also make those who believed it when the media and government immediately said it was a crazy conspiracy idea to think this was some kind of manmade virus released from a lab to think twice about who they should be believing.

Conspiracy idea #6 Alternative treatments are not effective or safe

Once again we have a topic that was so quickly set upon by the powers that be that one must be curious as to why. It seemed as though the moment that a cheap, easy, effective treatment may have been found to help save lives from the dreaded covid the government and the media would pounce on those who were revealing these options and denounce them as charlatans. Even the notion of intelligent debate regarding these possible solutions seemed to be forbidden. It seemed the only thing that was going to be accepted as safe and effective were new expensive pharmaceuticals and experimental vaccines.

The first of these alternative options to be revealed to the public was hydroxychloroquine(HCQ), made famous (or infamous) by President Trump announcing it as a "game changer" early on in 2020. Unfortunately, it was because of Trump's early support of hydroxychloroquine that led to its initial controversy and divisiveness as a potential therapy. Regardless that HCQ was a very cheap drug with a very long history of safe usage (72), if Trump supported something there was a very strong chance the media would immediately shut it down no matter if it was legitimate or not. This was exactly what happened with HCQ. Soon after Trump's support of HCQ came out, there were a few small papers being mentioned in the press that accused HCQ of creating potential heart problems; there was never any mention in these same press announcements that there had been far more research from before the pandemic that had already been published showing how HCQ could possibly help people with heart issues. (73) Instead there seemed to be a very quick judgment and indictment of HCQ. A year later in 2022, a paper in the European Journal of Epidemiology had this to say about the subject, "A timely completion of the remaining trials would have generated precise estimates of the potential effectiveness of HCQ to prevent COVID-19 among those at high risk of infection or complications. However, the widespread conviction about HCQ's lack of effectiveness dramatically slowed down the recruitment into ongoing trials of HCQ prophylaxis. As a result, key decisions were made based on insufficient evidence during the pre-vaccine period of the pandemic." (74) In other words, the rush to judgment over HCQ led to its demise as an effective treatment before it could even get started.

The next potential treatment that came up for summary judgment was Ivermectin (IVM). As early as April of 2020, there was already research coming out discussing the effectiveness of IVM with Covid-19 patients. (75) In July of 2020 a large group of doctors from India, "with vast experience in the management of Covid-19", gathered to evaluate IVM for its usage in the treatment of Covid-19. Citing current and on-going research, they concluded "that Ivermectin can be a potential molecule for prophylaxis and treatment of people infected with Coronavirus, owing to its anti-viral properties coupled with effective cost, availability and good tolerability and safety." (76) All told, there are close to a hundred studies showing some level of positive outcomes in the treatment of Covid-19 patients. (77) Despite this and despite the fact that IVM has a nearly flawless safety record over a very long period of usage and IVM is on the World Health Organization's List of Essential Medicines, the media and government agencies once again immediately pounced on anyone speaking out in favor of its usage (78,79,80) There was even a former W.H.O. consultant & research scientist, Tess Lawrie MD, PhD, who went on record stating that the evidence clearly showed the effectiveness of IVM for treatment of Covid-19 and that this information was being covered up. (81)

One very interesting point that people should understand when considering these facts is that the Government had initiated the Emergency Use Authorization (EUA) very early on in the pandemic. This act allows the creation of "unapproved medical products or unapproved uses of approved medical products to be used in an emergency to diagnose, treat, or prevent serious or life-threatening diseases or conditions caused by...threat agents when certain criteria are met, including there are no adequate, approved, and available alternatives."(82) The rules for the EUA are very clear and dictate that there can be "no adequate, approved, and available alternatives." As long as there was nothing available to treat Covid-19 that met these stipulations then the government and the pharmaceutical companies had carte blanche to create experimental vaccines and drugs as their remedy of choice. Another very important aspect to the EUA is that anything created while under its authorization is 100% protected from liability. You can not sue the pharmaceutical companies if you are injured or if a loved one dies from a product they create while under the EUA. And just so we are crystal clear, "Pfizer alone generated USD 35 billion net profits on its COVID-19 related products during 2021 and 2022. BioNTech and Moderna made USD 20 billion each, while Sinovac pocketed USD 15 billion." (83) Also, don't forget how intimately the government is involved with the pharmaceutical companies in this process. Our government spent heavily to promote the development of the vaccines, "estimates of direct public spending on the development and manufacturing of COVID-19 vaccines vary considerably based on the range of sources examined ... government spending estimates of between $18 billion and $23 billion." (84) Once again you need to ask yourself a serious question. Why were early treatments that were based on medications that were inexpensive and had long track records of safety summarily dismissed? And, Why then were brand new, expensive vaccines and drugs with no history for safety or effectiveness rushed into market and immediately and widely promoted and supported in their place? They can yell science (as long as it is their science), but I say follow the money.

Doctors who supported the usage of any of these "alternative" therapies were at great risk of losing their license to practice medicine. Prior to the pandemic, it was common practice to allow a doctor to treat their patients with the best methods that they saw fit. This was not something that was questioned unless there was negligence. During the pandemic however doctors were essentially told that there was one party line for treatment and if they went outside of this they would pay a price. Remember that this was a novel virus, which means a virus that has not affected humans before and therefore we do not really understand how to go about treating it. This should have meant more leeway to try treatments, not less. A great example of this were the doctors involved in Front Line Covid-19 Critical Care Alliance, Drs. Pierre Kory and Paul Marik, both of whom were ridiculed for treating patients with something other than the one approved protocol being dictated. (85) Both of these doctors lost their licenses as a result. (86)

Conspiracy idea #7 Anything said that even remotely went against the vaccines

We come at last to the pièce de résistance, the vaccines. Having read everything up to this final point, you will most likely not be surprised at the culmination of events leading up to this final piece of information. Even without the pandemic and all of the events leading up to and during it, this topic has always been a touchy one to say the least. As I have already mentioned previously, anyone who speaks out or even questions vaccines is immediately viewed as "anti-vaccine" and even "anti-science" and then unceremoniously canceled. This was even more evident during the pandemic. The vaccine apologists used the pandemic to infuse the vaccine topic with an even higher morality than ever before. You were either on board with the vaccine agenda or you were against it. There was no in between. If you supported the agenda you were for saving lives, if you asked questions or spoke out you were against saving lives. Doctors, celebrities or any citizen that spoke up was immediately ostracized. (87,88,89,90) A perfect example of how even an educated, respected voice against vaccines can lead to ridicule and attack by the media and the medical establishment is Dr Jessica Rose. Dr. Rose has an incredibly impressive list of accomplishments; she is a Canadian researcher with a Bachelor's Degree in

Applied Mathematics and a Master's degree in Immunology from Memorial University of Newfoundland. She also holds a PhD in Computational Biology from Bar Ilan University and 2 Post Doctoral degrees: one in Molecular Biology from the Hebrew University of Jerusalem and one in Biochemistry from the Technion Institute of Technology. She also has been a supporter of the vaccine program throughout her career, however when she began speaking out about concerns over the Covid vaccines she was immediately labeled an "anti-vaxxer" with a "history of spreading COVID-19 or vaccine misinformation." Another person (whom I already mentioned in the previous Point) with an equally impressive pedigree is Dr. Peter McCullough who is currently the Vice Chief of internal Medicine and Chief of Cardiovascular Research of the Baylor Heart and Vascular Institute. He serves as the Chief Academic and Scientific officer of the St. John Providence Health System. He holds a BS degree from Baylor University, a medical degree from the University of Texas Southwestern Medical School and a Master's in Public Health from the University of Michigan School of Public Health. His works have appeared in the *New England Journal of Medicine, Journal of the American Medical Association,* and other prestigious journals worldwide. Dr. McCullough has been an incredibly outspoken opponent of the covid vaccines and is also being mislabeled as a "spreader of misinformation" despite his long career of supporting the use of vaccines. (91, 92)

Even President Biden did his part in creating an environment of intolerance concerning this subject. "When asked what his message to platforms like Facebook regarding COVID-19 disinformation was, President Biden said: "I mean they really, look, the only pandemic we have is among the unvaccinated, and that's — they're killing people," he said during a press conference." (93) Nahid Bhadelia, MD, founding director of the Center for Emerging Infectious Diseases at Boston University agreed with the President's statement, "I think social media is playing a big role in amplifying misinformation, which is leading to people not taking the vaccine, which is killing them," Dr. Bhadelia said. "It's the honest truth. Covid, right now, is a vaccine-preventable disease." (93) Just for the record, both Anthony Fauci and President Biden contracted Covid after receiving not just the vaccine but also two booster shots. (94, 95) To add insult to injury, a study done at the Cleveland Clinic found that the risk of Covid-19 increased with the number of vaccines and boosters a person received. Not only did their study reveal this information but they also cited three other studies that reached the same conclusion as they did. (96) So much for Covid being "vaccine preventable."

Not only are the Covid vaccines not effective at preventing or stopping SARs-CoV-2, but they are the most dangerous vaccine that has ever been created. This may seem like a bold declaration yet when you look at the evidence to back up this statement you will see that it is not an exaggeration. At the time of this writing, the current data for reports regarding COVID vaccines to VAERS showed: 36,726 deaths, 212,294 hospitalizations, 17,575 Bell's palsy, 21,155 heart attacks, 27,832 myocarditis, 46,529 severe allergic reactions, 15,960 shingles and 68,819 permanently disabled.(97) To place a bit of perspective to these numbers all we need do is look at the number of deaths being reported since the introduction of the COVID vaccines. In about a three year time period we have a whopping 36,726 deaths being reported to VAERS. Compare this to the three years prior to the COVID vaccines and we only have 1,557 deaths. The simple fact that this obscene increase in the number of reported deaths has not created any concern among the purveyors of the vaccines is the truly alarming thing here. If this type of reporting had occurred with any other drug it would have immediately been pulled from circulation and the media would have been all over reporting it.

The fact is that the VAERS system was completely overwhelmed by the sheer volume of reports of issues from the COVID vaccines. This despite the CDC ramping up preparations to handle the increased amount of reporting from these new and experimental vaccines. The CDC , knowing that there would likely be an increase in VAERS reporting, contracted an outside source called General Dynamics Information Technology (GDIT) to help with the processing of the expected increase. The initial contract between the CDC and GDIT stated that "the total number of reports received during periods of peak activity is expected to be 1,000 reports per day, with up to 40%

of the reports serious in nature." (98) This alone is an alarming piece of information since the "1,000 reports per day" they were expecting is a nearly 700% increase from what would have been considered a normal amount of reports prior to the release of the COVID vaccines. Also the usual percentage of serious reports was closer to 5% not the 40% they were gearing up for. It truly begs the question of why the CDC was expecting the VAERS reporting to be so horrendous. What were they aware of that the public was not being told?

But wait, things get much worse. One month (January 15, 2021) into GDIT processing VAERS activity they wrote a report to the CDC stating, "Since release [of the vaccines] the number of incoming COVID-19 reports has significantly exceeded the estimated 1,000 reports per day. As a result, GDIT is unable to meet processing and other time frames." Up to the date above, GDIT states that they had received over 76,000 reports! This is in just the first month after the release of the COVID vaccines. By the time they produce their next report (February 2021) the number of reports for this next period has increased to 98,000! (98) During this same time frame the public was being told that the vaccines are safe, effective and that no harm is being reported. Just look at this one headline from April of 2021, "CDC Says It Has Seen No 'Signals' Linking COVID Vaccines and Myocarditis." (99) All one needs to do to see the lie is to look at the VAERS reporting system. In 2021, there were nearly 16,000 cases of myocarditis reported to VAERS and over 10,000 reported in 2022. (97) Even the Journal of the American Medical Association was reporting that "the risk of myocarditis after receiving mRNA-based COVID-19 vaccines was increased across multiple age and sex strata and was highest after the second vaccination dose in adolescent males and young men." They even went on to say, given the high verification rate of reports of myocarditis to VAERS after mRNA-based COVID-19 vaccination, underreporting is more likely. Therefore, the actual rates of myocarditis pre million doses of vaccine are likely higher than estimated." (100) The powers that be can lie and manipulate all they want but the facts are out there for those who wish to see them.

On top of increased risks for myocarditis, the COVID-19 vaccines have been linked to a plethora of other issues such as shingles, neurological and autoimmune conditions. (100,102,103,104,105) The larger concerns involve the long term usage of very experimental mRNA vaccines. A recent prospective cohort study compared vaccinated to unvaccinated 90 days after injection with a COVID-19 vaccine. The "rates of hematological abnormalities in the vaccination group 3 months after vaccination were significantly higher than those in the unvaccinated group." (106) The COVID-19 vaccines are the very first mRNA vaccines to be approved for usage and as such, we really do not understand what the possible long term outlook will be from continued injections with these vaccines. Scientists are far from agreement as to the long term safety of mRNA vaccines. (107,108,109,110) Yet the vaccine apologists want the world to know that these vaccines are perfectly safe and that we should not worry about them. With not one person from that side of the equation willing to even have an open and honest conversation involving the COVID-19 vaccines, how can we ever feel confident that the truth is being told? The sheer volume of lies, denials, half truths and slight-of-hand involving these vaccines can only lead one to believe that there is something nefarious going on. A very recent paper just came out of Italy and had incredibly damning evidence against the Covid vaccines. The authors went back and looked at a very large study done over a two year period in a province in Italy and compared those vaccinated with those unvaccinated from Covid to look at all cause deaths. What they found helps drive home the point I have been leading to. "We found all-cause death risks to be even higher for those vaccinated with one and two doses compared to the unvaccinated and that the booster doses were ineffective." (111) My real fear is that we are only scratching the surface of the damages these vaccines are causing to society.

The SARs-CoV-2 pandemic was seen by many people as simply a culmination of the efforts to control vaccine hesitancy that had already been building up over the years prior to 2020. If you have been adding up the information in all of the Points leading up to this one you may have noticed the pattern. Even if the origination of the virus is never confirmed or agreed upon, the actions that were taken after the virus began its spread are proof enough of a predetermined intent on the part of the vaccine apologists. The pandemic stands as a hallmark event in our history especially in regard to health freedom (possibly freedom in general). The decisions that were enacted during the pandemic are having and will have ongoing effects now and into the future. Freedoms once taken are difficult to regain. The old adage is incredibly true in this scenario: Those who do not learn from the past are doomed to repeat it.

Addendum:

On December 2, 2024, the Select Subcommittee on the Coronavirus Pandemic (a subcommittee of the House of Representatives Committee on Oversight and Accountability) released its final report after nearly two years of investigation. The committee included nine Republicans and seven Democrats. This document is over 500 pages of detailed information on many of the points I have already broken down in this chapter. I am adding this information as both an update and validation of the information already covered above. To date this is the most accurate breakdown of information brought forth regarding events during the Covid pandemic. (112)

The Sub Committee's report had a large number of findings, many of which I am not listing here. Those findings that relate directly (or closely) to the points I have made, or are otherwise relevant, are in bold (everything presented are direct quotes from the report):

SARS-CoV-2, the Virus that Causes COVID-19, Likely Emerged Because of a Laboratory or Research Related Accident.
Four years after the onset of the worst pandemic in 100 years, the weight of the evidence increasingly supports the lab leak hypothesis

"The Proximal Origin of SARS-CoV-2" Was "Prompted" by Dr. Anthony Fauci to "Disprove" the Lab Leak Theory.

There Was No Quantitative Scientific Support for Six Feet of Social Distancing.

- Social distancing requirements were largely responsible for closing businesses, heightening a sense in loss of community, and were part of the reasoning schools could not reopen for so long.
- The justification for one of the most impactful COVID-19 policies, that arguably affected the most Americans in their day-to-day lives, was "it sort of just appeared." There were no scientific trials or studies conducted before this policy was implemented, there

appeared to be no pushback or internal discussion amongst the highest level of leadership, and more importantly there appears to be no acceptance of responsibility

Masks and Mask Mandates Were Ineffective at Controlling the Spread of COVID19.

- A systematic review carried out by Cochrane Collaboration—one of the most highly regarded methodologies in evidence-based healthcare—found that the pooled randomized control trials they analyzed "did not show a clear reduction in respiratory viral infection with the use of medical/surgical masks"

Public Health Officials Flip Flopping on the Efficacy and Use of Face Masks Without Full Scientific Transparency Caused Mistrust in Public Health Establishments.

- During the COVID-19 pandemic, the worst public health crisis in our modern era, the CDC constantly redirected their opinions and provided conflicting answers. These actions undermined the American people's belief in the CDC, public health leadership, and science as a whole.

The Biden Administration Exceeded its Authority by Mandating Masks.

The U.S. Centers for Disease Control and Prevention Relied on Flawed Studies to Support the Issuance of Mask Mandates.

- In issuing guidances that mandated the use of masks across the country, the CDC publicly relied on several different studies to justify the actions. The CDC provided a list of approximately 15 studies that demonstrated wearing masks reduced new infections. Yet, all 15 of the provided studies are observational studies that were conducted after COVID-19 began and, importantly, none of them were RCTs.
- The trajectories of the rate of COVID-19 infections for states with mask mandates and states without is virtually identical.
- ItisapparentthattheCDCandtheBidenAdministration cherry-picked observational data to fit their narrative that masks are fully effective.

Forcibly Masking Young Children, Ages Two and Older, Caused More Harm than Good.

- Ignoring the science and facts of COVID-19 and the harms of masking young children was profoundly immoral on behalf of the leadership of the country's public health officials. The future consequences of these types of draconian policies are not yet known, but public health leaders in the future should remember that all policy must be decided in a balanced manner.

Enduring COVID-19 Lockdowns Unnecessarily Harmed the U.S. Economy.

Enduring COVID-19 Lockdowns Unnecessarily Damaged American's Mental Health.

Enduring COVID-19 Lockdowns Disrupted the Development of American Children and Young Adults.

Enduring COVID-19 Lockdowns Unnecessarily had Severe Consequences for Americans' Physical Health.

Public Health Officials Incorrectly Characterized the Lab-Leak Theory as a "Conspiracy Theory."

- During the early months of the pandemic, Dr. Fauci played a critical role in disparaging the lab-leak theory
- Dr. Fauci was also directly involved in the drafting and promotion of Proximal Origin, in which the authors concluded "we do not believe that any type of laboratory-based scenario is plausible." Evidence suggests that Dr. Fauci "prompted" the drafting of the Proximal Origin paper to "disprove" the lab-leak theory.

The Biden Administration Employed Undemocratic and Likely Unconstitutional Methods to Fight What It Deemed to Be Misinformation.

- An Interim Staff Report [hereinafter "Weaponization Report"], which highlighted some of the most egregious examples of the Biden White House's censorship campaign. The Judiciary Report found that major technology companies Meta, Alphabet, and Amazon changed their content moderation policies in response to pressure from the Biden White House.
- The White House led Facebook to take down posts which claimed that COVID-19 was "man-made, manufactured, bioengineered, a bioweapon, or created by an individual government or country, which includes claims that the virus was modified through gain of function research and leaked from a lab."
- The Judiciary Report also highlighted emails indicating that Biden White House officials pressured social media companies to take down or otherwise suppress posts related to other elements of the COVID-19 pandemic, including COVID-19 vaccines and therapeutics.

The Biden Administration and Many Public Health Officials Exaggerated the Power of COVID-19 Vaccines.

- On more than one occasion, President Biden himself overstated the vaccine's ability to prevent infection and transmission. These false statements likely contributed to Americans' confusion about COVID-19 vaccines and reduced overall vaccine confidence.

- During his announcement of the COVID-19 vaccine mandate for federal workers and contractors on September 9, 2021, President Biden implied that COVID-19 vaccines were effective at preventing the spread of the virus when he said, "The bottom line – we're going to protect vaccinated workers from unvaccinated coworkers."

- Other officials also made false or misleading statements about COVID-19 vaccines. On March 29, 2021, during an appearance on the Rachel Maddow Show, Dr. Walensky claimed that CDC data indicated that "vaccinated people do not carry the virus, don't get sick, and that it's not just in the clinical trials but its also in the real-world data."On May 16, 2021, during an appearance on CBS' Face the Nation, Dr. Fauci claimed that vaccinated individuals can go without masks even if they have an asymptomatic case of COVID19 because "it is very unlikely that a vaccinated person, even if there's a breakthrough infection, would transmit it to someone else." Dr. Fauci also took it a step further and indicated that vaccinated people become "dead ends" for the virus.

- Even with the most charitable read of the contemporary data supporting these statements, it appears these were gross overstatements of the COVID-19 vaccines' protective abilities, even against the earlier variants.

- Perhaps conveniently, the CDC stopped tracking all breakthrough infections beginning May 1, 2021, and instead only tracked breakthrough cases that led to hospitalization or death. The CDC argued that this decision would help "maximize the quality of the data collected on cases of greatest clinical and public health importance." The CDC's final report showing breakthrough infections indicated that 10,262 infections had occurred across 46 U.S. states.

The U.S. Food and Drug Administration and Other Public Health Officials Falsely Implied that Ivermectin Was Only for Horses and Cows

- One of the most egregious examples of the Biden Administration's purveyance of misinformation—the FDA's infamous statement which implied that Ivermectin was a veterinary drug for horses and cows and not for humans.
- The Biden Administration Sidelined Senior Scientists After They Expressed Concern Regarding the Rapid Pace of Review of Pfizer's Biologics Approval Application.

The Biden Administration Accelerated the Approval of Pfizer's Biologics Approval Application to Impose Vaccine Mandates

- It is highly concerning that paving the way for mandatory vaccination policies played any role at all in the FDA's process for approving COVID-19 vaccines, and even worse that it appears to have played a primary role in their rationale for casting aside top vaccine experts and hyper-accelerating the target date

Herd Immunity is a Real Concept and Occurrence Supported by Public Health Leaders, Such as Dr. Fauci, and There Was a Coordinated Effort from Public Health Officials to Ignore Natural Immunity and Suppress Dissenting Opinions.

- Many researchers recognized the existing science and called for policy makers and government officials to use infection acquired immunity from COVID-19 to help control the spread of virus. Many countries around the world allowed a previous COVID-19 infection to satisfy the individual's "vaccination status." Yet U.S. public health officials resisted including infection acquired immunity when developing guidance and policy during the pandemic.

- The Great Barrington Declaration was an open letter published in October 2020 in response to mass lockdowns. Originally signed by scientists from the University of Oxford, Stanford University, and Harvard University, the document presented the idea that lockdowns had adverse effects on both the mental and physical health of populations. It called for a "focused protection" pandemic strategy

- Critics of this idea immediately disqualified the proposal, to an unsettling degree never seen before in the scientific community. Anyone associated with the paper was immediately categorized as a "fringe" theorist. Rather than being allowed to engage in scientific and political debate, the alternative proposal was dubbed dangerous and referred to as a "let it rip," meaning the vast spread of the virus, approach.

- This kind of rhetoric and behavior created a scientific environment that fostered hostility and outright contempt for differing opinions. Scientists and doctors were demonized by colleagues and peers within their own community.

COVID-19 Vaccine Mandates Caused Massive Collateral Damage and Were Very Likely Counterproductive.

- Vaccines alone, and therefore COVID-19 vaccine mandates, could not and did not bring us to "herd immunity." Yet, they caused collateral damage that has been felt by millions of Americans.
- COVID-19 vaccine mandates also forced millions of people to choose between their livelihoods and being vaccinated—even if they had closely held personal or religious beliefs or a medical reason. This is not only unjust, but it also caused thousands of people to lose their jobs in the middle of a pandemic and unstable economic environment.

COVID-19 Vaccine Mandates Were Not Supported by Science.

- The COVID-19 vaccine mandates applied a one-size-fits-all approach to medicine which seriously undermined the patient-physician relationship.

COVID-19 Vaccine Mandates Hampered U.S. Military Readiness.

- According to reports, only 43 of the more than 8,000 separated service members rejoined the military. The DOD COVID-19 vaccine mandate directly led to the separation of thousands of US service members, but it has also hindered the military's ability to recruit.

The Vaccine Adverse Event Reporting System is Insufficient and Not Transparent.

- Anyone can submit a report to VAERS, and these reports are automatically published and available publicly. Therefore, a report on VAERS has likely not been proven to be caused by a vaccine. However, the vast discrepancy when comparing COVID19 vaccines over three years, with all other vaccines over more than 30 years raises serious concerns.

Existing Vaccine Safety Systems May Be Missing Important Safety Signals, Especially Related to Neurological Conditions.

The U.S. Centers for Disease Control and Prevention Created a New Surveillance System Specifically for COVID-19 but has not been Fully Transparent in Sharing the Data Collected in it

- According to CDC, 10.1 million V-Safe participants completed more than 151 million surveys about their health experiences after receiving COVID-19 and mpox vaccines.
- ICAN obtained and released the "checkbox" data in October 2022. ICAN also created a public dashboard which highlights the data, which they say contains "numerous alarming results." Specifically, ICAN reports that the data show 782,913 individuals, or more than 7.7 percent of users, reported a health event requiring medical attention, emergency room intervention, and/or hospitalization.

A Robust and Transparent Vaccine Injury Compensation Program Is Necessary for Promoting Trust in Vaccines.

Debating or Discussing Vaccine Injury Compensation Is Not "Anti-Vax," and Implications Otherwise Are Counterproductive to Protecting Public Health.

- This divisive language was a critical misstep of the COVID-19 vaccination campaign which alienated and dismissed people who had experienced rare but life-altering adverse reactions to the vaccine.

Pandemic-Era Policy Often Disregarded or Outright Violated the Sanctity of the Doctor-Patient Relationship

The Use of Off-Label Prescriptions Was Unjustly Demonized and Further Eroded the Doctor-Patient Relationship.

- During the pandemic, the off-label uses of possible treatments for COVID-19 were swiftly and systematically demonized. Doctors frequently reprimanded, threatened, censored, or even fired by their employers for doing so. The federal government weaponized public health agencies to promote fear surrounding drugs such as Ivermectin and Hydroxychloroquine.

The Final Point

I honestly believe that the vaccine program began from a good place. Those that were there at the beginning of the vaccine program in the 1900's saw disease and death all around them and wanted to help protect us. They put their collective brains to use and came up with vaccines as a way to create this protection. I find this admirable. The problem is that even the best of intentions can go awry.

The vaccine program now is not remotely the vaccine program that was begun back then. The changes to this program became glaring after 1986 and have only gotten worse. Not only are we dealing with an exponentially larger number of doses of antigens, adjuvants and by-products being injected into our children, we are also now dealing with a program that not only has zero liability, but has been completely captured by the same companies responsible for making the products that have zero liability. The inmates are in charge of the asylum.

If this were not bad enough, those that are in charge of every step of this entire program seem to have no real care for truth. They seem to have no real concern for anything other than their collective bottom line, whether that is money, power, control or some misguided belief that everything really is a-okay is unclear. What is crystal clear is that there are a multitude of issues/problems with this program that need to be solved before it continues to make things worse. The problems that need to be addressed would include:

1. Who is running the "hen house?" The agencies that are supposed to be looking out for us are instead looking out for themselves and the pharmaceutical companies. Money and jobs rotate in and out

of the companies and agencies like a merry go round. Corporate capture is rampant. There is NO real oversight.

2. Who is held responsible? The pharmaceutical companies have NO liability for their vaccines doing harm (short term or long term). ALL of the other products they make have some level of liability on them and therefore there is some incentive to create products that are "safe." However, even with this liability these same companies regularly put products on the market that harm or kill people, often times (proven) knowingly. When there is zero liability on vaccines there is zero responsibility.

3. What about the children? We now have the sickest generation of kids in American history. Instead of going through even more of the research to back this claim up I will refer you to an excellent article written by Children's Health Defense. (https://childrenshealthdefense.org/news/chronically-ill-children-who-is-sounding-the-alarm/)They have already done an excellent job presenting this information so I will not attempt to improve upon what they have already done. The one point I will mention here is that studies have shown that over half of American children now have some type of chronic disease. The big question that is not being addressed (more like swept under the rug) is why? The vaccine apologists refuse to look at vaccines as a possible causative agent. They insist that there is no way vaccines could be linked to anything like this. They make this claim with NO research to conclusively prove their point. They do not want to prove this point because if (or when) the truth is revealed regarding the harm from vaccines, their entire stack of cards will come crumbling down. The capture of our media.

4. The capture of our media. Although not strictly part of the vaccine issue, it is through the lens of the vaccine issue that the capture of our media becomes so apparent. Our media is following the orders of their major advertisers, the pharmaceutical companies. When 75% of T.V. ads are coming from the pharmaceutical companies it should be easy to see how they are running the show.

Any messaging that harms the pharma cartel will result in advertising dollars being removed. This ensures compliance from the media and results in a clearly controlled message that eliminates unwanted questions and negativity regarding vaccines. Eliminating direct-to-consumer advertising of medical products (just like all but two countries in the entire world already do) would be a great leap forward to removing this obstacle.

5. Freedom of choice! The final piece to this issue is giving back full freedom of choice when it comes to an individual's medical decisions. As more and more states remove the philosophical exemption from existence our freedom of choice rapidly diminishes. The philosophical exemption is the only one of the three exemptions that is truly based on freedom of choice. This exemption merely states that the individual can "just say no." This is what true freedom of choice should be all about. The religious and medical exemptions leave a lot of control still in regulators hands so that they can still deny us our right to choose. Our bodies, our health. The government (and the pharmaceutical companies that have so much influence) should not be able to force anyone to inject themselves against their will (period).

With all of that said, I should make clear that the term "anti-vaxxer" does not really resonate with me. It is not a matter of being completely against the idea of vaccines, but instead I am against the way this vaccine program IS. The number of issues, problems and other questionables related to the current vaccine program is overwhelming and a huge problem that needs to be addressed. Safety, accountability, transparency, corruption, trust, honesty, and so much more are the issues. The idea of something (perhaps a vaccine) that could save or protect us from dangers is not (to me) a crazy idea. So from that perspective, I am not "anti-vaccine." However, in its current form and with the current people running the show, I am completely "anti this vaccine program." While I have far more trust in the power of my own body than outside chemical agents, if it were possible to create a truly safe product that could help save lives from deadly diseases AND if the power to choose to take or not take this product was left intact, then I suppose I would be alright with the idea. This is certainly not the way things currently stand. Until the day the issues listed above are fully addressed the vaccine program as it exists currently is untrustworthy and dangerous. The more individuals become educated to the actual facts regarding the vaccine program the greater the likelihood for these changes to take place can eventually become a reality. I encourage everyone who reads this book to take the extra time to look at the research cited within these pages and take ownership of the information. Don't just take my words here as the truth, instead double check everything I have written and then trust your own mind as to the integrity of this information.

"You can either be informed and your own rulers, or you can be ignorant and have someone else, who is not ignorant, rule over you."
~ Julian Assange

Or perhaps

"There must be a happy medium somewhere between being totally informed and blissfully unaware."
~ Doug Larson

Educational Material

Books:

- *A Shot in the Dark* by Harris L. Coulter and Barbara Loe Fisher
- *The Vaccine Guide: Risks and Benefits for Children and Adults* by Randall Neustaedter
- *Miller's Review of Critical Vaccine Studies* by Neil Z. Miller
- *Dissolving Illusions: Disease, Vaccines and the Forgotten History* by Suzanne Humphries, MD and Roman Bystrianyk
- *Callous Disregard: Autism and Vaccines--The Truth Behind a Tragedy* by Andrew J. Wakefield
- *The Age of Autism: Mercury, Medicine, and a Man-Made Epidemic* by Dan Olmsted
- *Vaccine Epidemic: How Corporate Greed, Biased Science, and Coercive Government Threaten Our Human Rights, Our Health, and Our Children* by Louise Kuo Habakus, Mary Holland
- *The HPV Vaccine on Trial: Seeking Justice for a Generation Betrayed* by Mary Holland, Kim Mack Rosenberg, et al.
- *Saying No to Vaccines: A Resource Guide for All Ages* by Dr. Sherri Tenpenny
- *The Environmental and Genetic Causes of Autism* by James
- Lyons-Weiler, PhD
- *Cures Vs. Profits: Successes In Translational Research* by James
- Lyons-Weiler
- *Vax-Unvax: Let the Science Speak* by Robert F. Kennedy Jr. and Brian Hooker PhD
- *Thimerosal: Let the Science Speak: The Evidence Supporting the Immediate Removal of Mercury—a Known Neurotoxin—from Vaccines* by Robert F. Kennedy Jr. , Mark Hyman, et al. | Sep 1, 2015
- *How to Raise a Healthy Child in Spite of Your Doctor* by Robert S. Mendelsohn, MD
- *Turtles All The Way Down: Vaccine Science and Myth,* by Anonymous (Author), Zoey O'Toole (Editor), Mary Holland J.D. (Editor, Foreword)

- *The Real Anthony Fauci* by Robert F. Kennedy Jr.
- *Follow the Science* by Sharyl Attkisson
- *The Pfizer Papers* by Naomi Wolf
- *Vaccines, Amen: The Religion of Vaccines* by Aaron Siri

Media:

- https://thehighwire.com/
- https://childrenshealthdefense.org/
- https://sharylattkisson.com/
- https://greenmedinfo.com/
- https://medscienceresearch.com/
- https://www.nvic.org/
- https://learntherisk.org/
- https://www.darksidevaccines.com/
- https://publichealthpolicyjournal.com/
- https://thecausesofautism.com/
- https://howdovaccinescauseautism.org/

Movies:

- Vaxxed, Vaxxed II and Vaxxed III
  https://vaxxedthemovie.com/
- The Greater Good
  https://greatergoodmovie.org/
- A Shot in the Dark
  https://archive.org/details/a-shot-in-the-dark-2020-documentary-vaccines-murder-and-mame
- Vaccination the Hidden Truth
  https://archive.org/details/Vaccination..The.Hidden.Truth.1998
- The Bought Movie
  https://www.kindearth.net/the-bought-movie-watch-free-online-essential-viewing/
- Deadly Immunity
  https://archive.org/details/deadly-immunity-by-robert-f.-kennedy-jr.
- An Inconvenient Study
  https://www.aninconvenientstudy.com/

References

References for Point Number One

1. https://pubmed.ncbi.nlm.nih.gov/26675613/.
2. https://depts.washington.edu/bhdept/ethics-medicine/bioethics-topics/articles/principles-bioethics
3. https://www.nejm.org/doi/full/10.1056/nejm199711133372006
4. https://www.foxnews.com/media/alan-dershowitz-forced-coronavirus-vaccinations-are-constitutional
5. https://www.sss.gov/conscientious-objectors/
6. https://www.nvic.org/Vaccine-Laws/state-vaccine-requirements.aspx
7. https://www.ncsl.org/research/health/school-immunization-exemption-state-laws.aspx
8. https://www.globalcitizen.org/en/content/esto-es-lo-que-necesitas-saber-sobre-la-nueva-ley/
9. https://hslda.org/post/bill-to-let-11-year-olds-make-medical-decision-will-congress-say-no
10. https://www.ksby.com/news/california-news/a-new-ca-bill-could-allow-12-to-17-year-olds-to-get-vaccinated-without-parental-consent

References for Point Number Two

1. https://www.vox.com/2014/10/13/6957875/christopher-columbus-murderer-tyrant-scoundrel
2. https://www.insider.com/us-history-facts-not-true-2019-4#myth-the-first-thanksgiving-was-a-peaceful-and-joyous-meal-shared-between-the-pilgrims-and-native-americans-4
3. *Dissolving Illusions*, by Suzanne Humphries, MD and Roman Bystrianyk
4. https://www.cdc.gov/mmwr/preview/mmwrhtml/mm4829a1.htm
5. https://www.history.com/topics/middle-ages/black-death
6. https://www.ncbi.nlm.nih.gov/pmc/articles/PMC4373148/

7. The Questionable Contribution of Medical Measures to the Decline of Mortality in the United States in the Twentieth Century on JSTOR
8. https://www.sciencedirect.com/science/article/pii/S0264410X17308551?via%3Dihub
9. https://pubmed.ncbi.nlm.nih.gov/24330942/
10. https://www.ncbi.nlm.nih.gov/pmc/articles/PMC2677258/#:~:text=For%20infectious%20diseases%20where%20immunization,asymptomatic%20encounters%20with%20the%20infection.
11. https://www.medscape.com/answers/300455-107822/what-is-the-mortality-and-morbidity-of-measles-virus-pneumonia

References for Point Number 3

1. https://www.csiro.au/en/Research/OandA/Areas/Assessing-our-climate/Climate-change-QA/Science
2. https://www.statista.com/statistics/686906/pharma-ad-spend-usa/
3. https://law.hofstra.edu/pdf/academics/journals/lawreview/lrv_issues_v35n02_dd7_lipman_final.pdf
4. https://centerforhealthjournalism.org/2017/06/16/conflicts-interest-health-care-journalism-who%E2%80%99s-watching-watchdogs-we-are-part-1-3
5. https://www.rollingstone.com/culture/culture-features/anti-vaxxers-facebook-youtube-instagram-806504/
6. https://www.cnbc.com/2019/05/20/alphabet-verily-doing-clinical-trials-with-novartis-sanofi-pfizer.html
7. https://www.cnbc.com/2019/02/21/fda-head-says-federal-government-may-take-action-if-states-dont-adjust-lax-vaccine-exemption-laws.html
8. https://www.cdc.gov/mmwr/preview/mmwrhtml/00041753.htm
9. https://www.ncbi.nlm.nih.gov/pmc/articles/PMC1522578/
10. https://www.constituteproject.org/constitution/United_States_of_America_1992

11. https://nypost.com/2021/02/19/white-house-working-with-social-media-to-silence-anti-vaxxers/?utm_source=facebook&utm_medium=news_tab&utm_content=algorithm&fbclid=IwAR2v6-yrYWyiLmTwbmhs_gPyg4WclVS1r9xs-NOl-YC0Pl0NXPBQZb3e5Kwc
12. https://www.sevenstories.com/books/3302-media-control
13. https://www.scientificamerican.com/article/how-the-fda-manipulates-the-media/
14. https://www.nytimes.com/2020/04/09/business/coronavirus-health-workers-speak-out.html
15. https://www.bostonglobe.com/2021/04/30/nation/celebrity-doctor-maine-blocked-instagram-over-covid-19-vaccine-misinformation-claims/
16. https://www.foxnews.com/media/minnesota-doctors-silenced-covid-views-masks-natural-immunity-vaccines
17. https://www.nytimes.com/2021/08/27/technology/doctors-virus-misinformation.html
18. https://www.latimes.com/business/story/2021-08-16/doctors-coronavirus-misinformation-license
19. https://www.cbc.ca/news/canada/british-columbia/bc-doctors-misinformation-covid-19-1.6021489
20. https://www.westernjournal.com/key-scientist-behind-mrna-vaccines-kicked-off-twitter-speaking-covid-vax/
21. https://www.nbcnews.com/think/opinion/eric-clapton-s-covid-vaccine-conspiracies-mark-sad-final-act-ncna1281619
22. https://uproxx.com/movies/evangeline-lilly-marvel-anti-vaxx-simu-liu/
23. https://www.vanityfair.com/hollywood/2022/01/marvel-star-evangeline-lilly-attended-anti-vaccine-mandate-protest

References for Point Number Four

1. https://www.hrsa.gov/vaccine-compensation/index.html
2. https://www.ncbi.nlm.nih.gov/books/NBK236419/
3. https://www.gao.gov/assets/670/667136.pdf
4. https://digital.ahrq.gov/sites/default/files/docs/publication/r18hs017045-lazarus-final-report-2011.pdf

5. https://www.cnn.com/2019/01/31/health/purdue-pharma-unredacted-lawsuit/index.html?utm_medium=social&utm_source=fbCNN&utm_content=2019-02-01T16:53:08&fbclid=IwAR0Zl36S38L94JgBeCQ_6C6hDwzMeezxjKTZ1Lu669zA1nQ6vwgu8XrGQRM
6. https://www.justice.gov/opa/pr/us-pharmaceutical-company-merck-sharp-dohme-sentenced-connection-unlawful-promotion-vioxx
7. https://www.npr.org/2007/11/10/5470430/timeline-the-rise-and-fall-of-vioxx
8. https://www.cbsnews.com/news/merck-created-hit-list-to-destroy-neutralize-or-discredit-dissenting-doctors/
9. https://www.pharmaceutical-technology.com/features/biggest-pharmaceutical-lawsuits/
10. https://www.enjuris.com/blog/resources/largest-pharmaceutical-settlements-lawsuits/
11. https://florinroebig.com/class-action/pharmaceutical/
12. https://www.nasdaq.com/press-release/tamiflu-fraud-bilked-%241.5-billion-from-government-alleges-whistleblower-2020-01-13?fbclid=IwAR0PkVmb_pwbSVzP5eF5fplXNuC6mmM3727zbuVC-cqJR_HkVp-sL25LZiE
13. https://www.marketsandmarkets.com/PressReleases/vaccine-technologies.asp?fbclid=IwAR3h0abgM-exGptE3i2n17OQMWIl5CZt75gU-l-sAVN0Dnn599Z6DPxW6wE
14. https://www.sec.gov/news/press/2011/2011-87.htm
15. https://www.theguardian.com/us-news/2019/sep/11/pfas-toxic-forever-chemicals-hearing-3m-dupont-chemours
16. https://www.drugwatch.com/featured/clinical-trials-and-hidden-data/
17. https://www.businessinsider.com/lawmakers-bought-sold-covid-19-related-stocks-during-pandemic-2021-12

References for Point Number Five

1. https://www.ncbi.nlm.nih.gov/pmc/articles/PMC1805729/
2. https://pubmed.ncbi.nlm.nih.gov/10578674/
3. https://pubmed.ncbi.nlm.nih.gov/12775615/
4. https://www.ncbi.nlm.nih.gov/pmc/articles/PMC3341407/

5. https://www.ncbi.nlm.nih.gov/pmc/articles/PMC1140949/
6. https://www.ncbi.nlm.nih.gov/pmc/articles/PMC5696751/
7. https://www.bbc.com/news/science-environment-39054778
8. https://www.salon.com/2014/01/25/5_evil_ways_the_multi_billion_dollar_drug_industry_is_in_bed_with_your_doctor_partner/
9. http://www.whale.to/drugs/fda.html
10. https://www.sciencemag.org/news/2018/07/hidden-conflicts-pharma-payments-fda-advisers-after-drug-approvals-spark-ethical
11. https://www.ncbi.nlm.nih.gov/pmc/articles/PMC1450069/
12. https://www.drugwatch.com/manufacturers/
13. https://www.ncbi.nlm.nih.gov/pmc/articles/PMC7054854/#:~:text=Pharmaceutical%20and%20health%20product%20industry%20spending%20on,averaged%20%24233%20million%20per%20year.
14. https://pubmed.ncbi.nlm.nih.gov/24088146/
15. https://apnews.com/article/9b72ea1408f-845eaa26638a652df2912
16. https://finance.yahoo.com/news/congress-big-pharma-money-123757664.html?guce_referrer=aHR0cHM6Ly93d3cuZ29vZ2xlLmNvbS8&guce_referrer_sig=AQAAAHz2RxkgGeCtZSo-b_27YiUEZ9DINnQFCAZORkm_czJYssj38T-LUSP7JWS8r_2s8XhgjdJQ7TfX3nq8n6h9JsgmjbEP2Dqbk-8WKGhhWazxeUDQ951OY-X-J3ooi5EcMXp-ABEg-kSXU-LobdYWUFhP2QWaJZUDr3evahzY8fmg0Iq&fbclid=IwAR1-Y_ZseTr13PK5sZ7nytCp_O5RiwSPjtwUr9jxEbXrMLRkx-0A7I_5O8krc&_guc_consent_skip=1648585497
17. https://rooseveltinstitute.org/2019/05/22/capturing-the-government-big-pharmas-take-over-of-policymaking/
18. https://rooseveltinstitute.org/wp-content/uploads/2020/07/RI_Pharma_Cost-of-Capture_brief_201905.pdf
19. https://www.washingtonpost.com/investigations/senators-call-for-crack-down-on-pharmaceutical-industry-revolving-door/2017/11/02/d0c3e6a2-bf34-11e7-959c-fe2b598d8c00_story.html

20. https://thehill.com/blogs/congress-blog/politics/452654-for-big-pharma-the-revolving-door-keeps-spinning
21. https://en.wikipedia.org/wiki/Michael_R._Taylor
22. https://wallmine.com/people/5297/julie-l-gerberding
23. https://khn.org/news/big-pharma-greets-hundreds-of-ex-federal-workers-at-the-revolving-door/
24. https://rooseveltinstitute.org/wp-content/uploads/2020/07/RI_Pharma_Cost-of-Capture_brief_201905.pdf
25. https://www.bmj.com/content/354/bmj.i5055
26. https://www.lawfirms.com/resources/environment/environment-health/cdc-members-own-more-50-patents-connected-vaccinations
27. https://patents.justia.com/assignee/centers-for-disease-control-and-prevention?page=10
28. https://www.cdc.gov/vaccines/imz-managers/guides-pubs/downloads/vacc_mandates_chptr13.pdf
29. https://www.govinfo.gov/content/pkg/CHRG-106hhrg73042/html/CHRG-106hhrg73042.htm
30. https://www.nytimes.com/2009/12/18/health/policy/18cdc.html
31. https://thehill.com/blogs/pundits-blog/healthcare/301432-the-cdc-is-being-being-influenced-by-corporate-and-political
32. https://www.prnewswire.com/news-releases/cdc-blocks-testimony-of-vaccine-whistleblower-says-world-mercury-project-300347376.html
33. https://www.euronews.com/health/2023/02/03/how-is-the-world-health-organization-funded-and-why-does-it-rely-so-much-on-bill-gates
34. https://archive.globalpolicy.org/home/270-general/52830-who-do-financial-contributions-from-pharma-violate-who-guidelines.html
35. https://pmc.ncbi.nlm.nih.gov/articles/PMC8202098/
36. https://citeseerx.ist.psu.edu/document?repid=rep1&type=pdf&doi=b59032c11ab7db60f40e9842dc2e9abe9198252f
37. https://childrenshealthdefense.org/wp-content/uploads/Godlee-2010-Conflicts-of-interest-and-pandemic-flu.pdf
38. https://www.bmj.com/content/340/bmj.c641

39. https://www.bmj.com/content/340/bmj.c3033
40. https://www.politico.com/news/2022/09/14/global-covid-pandemic-response-bill-gates-partners-00053969
41. https://www.modernatx.com/en-US/partnerships/strategic-collaborators
42. https://jamanetwork.com/journals/jama/fullarticle/2770485
43. https://www.youtube.com/watch?v=038__DssSv0&t=3270s
44. https://www.clarkcountytoday.com/news/pfizer-vaccine-bonanza-slows-but-bill-gates-sold-early-made-huge-profits/
45. https://www.who.int/news-room/detail/04-09-2019-vaccine-misinformation-statement-by-who-director-general-on-facebook-and-instagram
46. https://expose-news.com/2022/10/30/youtube-announces-partnership-with-who/
47. https://www.businessinsider.com/who-wuhan-scientists-initially-worried-coronavirus-leaked-lab-2021-3
48. https://www.dailymail.co.uk/news/article-10099969/Third-World-Health-Organizations-team-investigating-Covids-origins-conflicts-interest.html
49. https://www.wsj.com/articles/covid-origin-china-lab-leak-807b7b0a
50. https://www.wsj.com/articles/fbi-director-says-covid-pandemic-likely-caused-by-chinese-lab-leak-13a5e69b

References for Point 6

1. https://www.frontiersin.org/journals/immunology/articles/10.3389/fimmu.2024.1509379/full
2. https://www.cnbc.com/2019/02/21/fda-head-says-federal-government-may-take-action-if-states-dont-adjust-lax-vaccine-exemption-laws.html
3. https://www.nejm.org/doi/10.1056/NEJM198703263161303
4. https://www.cdc.gov/measles/about/history.html
5. https://pubmed.ncbi.nlm.nih.gov/1884314/.
6. https://academic.oup.com/jid/article/207/6/990/898747
7. https://pubmed.ncbi.nlm.nih.gov/24585562/
8. https://www.cdc.gov/mmwr/preview/mmwrhtml/mm6438a7.htm

9. https://jcm.asm.org/content/jcm/55/3/735.full.pdf
10. https://www.latimes.com/local/california/la-me-ln-whooping-cough-vaccine-20190316-story.html
11. https://www.nejm.org/doi/full/10.1056/NEJM199407073310104
12. https://www.cidrap.umn.edu/news-perspective/2019/06/whooping-cough-cases-tied-waning-vaccine-protection
13. https://pubmed.ncbi.nlm.nih.gov/26987576/
14. https://pubmed.ncbi.nlm.nih.gov/19815120/
15. https://pubmed.ncbi.nlm.nih.gov/18444852/
16. https://pubmed.ncbi.nlm.nih.gov/5117594/
17. https://academic.oup.com/cid/article/56/10/1363/404283?login=true
18. https://www.cdc.gov/mmwr/preview/mmwrhtml/mm6342a3.htm?s_cid=mm6342a3_e
19. https://pubmed.ncbi.nlm.nih.gov/1679866/
20. https://www.sciencedirect.com/science/article/pii/S0264410X18304857?via%3Dihub#bb0055

References for Point Number Seven

1. https://www.merriam-webster.com/dictionary/safe
2. https://www.aafp.org/news/media-center/kits/vaccines-are-safe-effective-and-save-lives.html
3. https://www.unicef.org/parenting/health/parents-frequently-asked-questions-vaccines
4. https://www.nationalacademies.org/based-on-science/vaccines-are-safe
5. https://www.cdc.gov/vaccines/parents/why-vaccinate/vaccine-decision.html
6. https://www.who.int/news-room/questions-and-answers/item/vaccines-and-immunization-what-is-vaccination
7. https://www.supremecourt.gov/opinions/10pdf/09-152.pdf
8. https://www.congress.gov/106/crpt/hrpt977/CRPT-106hrpt977.pdf
9. https://www.historyofvaccines.org/timeline#EVT_24
10. https://www.ncbi.nlm.nih.gov/pmc/articles/PMC2376879/
11. https://www.ncbi.nlm.nih.gov/books/NBK234365/

12. https://www.ncbi.nlm.nih.gov/books/NBK225459/
13. https://www.nature.com/articles/1206547
14. https://europepmc.org/abstract/med/7473072
15. https://books.google.com/books?hl=en&lr=&id=J_qbAgAAQBAJ&oi=fnd&pg=PR1&dq=sv40+and+cancer+-studies&ots=PnC5koDkQ2&sig=dAozaRWoZPYqlRV8gp-FNxAgAFTk#v=onepage&q=sv40%20and%20cancer%20studies&f=false
16. https://www.ncbi.nlm.nih.gov/pmc/articles/PMC2965816/
17. https://www.ncbi.nlm.nih.gov/pubmed/552571/
18. https://www.ncbi.nlm.nih.gov/pmc/articles/PMC4494348/
19. https://www.ema.europa.eu/en/documents/variation-report/pandemrix-H-c-832-ii-0061-epar-assessment-report-variation_en.pdf
20. .https://www.mctlaw.com/101-million-dollar-vaccine-injury-mmr/
21. https://www.ncbi.nlm.nih.gov/pmc/articles/PMC5360569/pdf/main.pdf
22. https://www.bmj.com/content/355/bmj.i5170.long
23. https://vaccinelaw.com/lawyer/2018/05/24/Vaccine-Injury/What-are-the-Most-Common-Vaccine-Injuries_bl34405.htm#:~:-text=Adhesive%20capsulitis%20(frozen%20shoulder),Shoulder%20bursitis
24. https://www.vaccineinjurylegalteam.com/news-information/vaccine-injury-information/
25. https://www.hrsa.gov/sites/default/files/vaccinecompensation/vaccineinjurytable.pdf
26. https://www.nap.edu/read/1815/chapter/2
27. https://www.nia.nih.gov/health/placebos-clinical-trials
28. https://www.clinicaltrials.gov/ct2/show/NCT00004800
29. https://www.fda.gov/media/77017/download
30. https://www.sciencedirect.com/science/article/abs/pii/S014067368191847X
31. https://link.springer.com/article/10.1186/s13054-017-1601-9
32. .https://www.sciencedirect.com/science/article/abs/pii/S0140673615603105
33. https://www.nejm.org/doi/full/10.1056/NEJM199510193331604

34. https://www.ncbi.nlm.nih.gov/pmc/articles/PMC4157320/
35. https://www.nature.com/articles/s41467-020-18305-y
36. https://vaers.hhs.gov/about.html
37. https://rickjaffeesq.com/wp-content/uploads/2021/02/r18hs017045-lazarus-final-repor t-20116.pdf
38. https://www.hrsa.gov/vaccine-compensation/about/index.html
39. https://www.cdc.gov/vaccinesafety/ensuringsafety/monitoring/vaers/reportingaes.html#:~:text=The%20VICP%20compensates%20people%20whose,for%20compensation%20with%20the%20VICP.
40. https://www.nvic.org/PDFs/ACCV/BanyonReport-VICPResearchReport.aspx
41. https://www.hrsa.gov/sites/default/files/hrsa/vaccine-compensation/data/vicp-stats-03-01-22.pdf
42. https://pubmed.ncbi.nlm.nih.gov/26021988/
43. Vaccines and sudden infant death: An analysis of the VAERS database 1990–2019 and review of the medical literature - ScienceDirect
44. https://www.ncbi.nlm.nih.gov/pmc/articles/PMC1647245/pdf/amjph00259-0017.pdf
45. https://pubmed.ncbi.nlm.nih.gov/6835859/
46. https://journals.lww.com/amjforensicmedicine/fulltext/2019/09000/sudden_infant_death_after_vaccination__survey_of.5.aspx
47. https://www.ncbi.nlm.nih.gov/pmc/articles/PMC1505512/pdf/bmjcred00658-0031.pdf
48. https://ecf.cofc.uscourts.gov/cgi-bin/show_public_doc?2013vv0611-73-0
49. https://www.researchgate.net/publication/271081102_Serum_antibodies_from_epileptic_patients_react_at_high_prevalence_with_simian_virus_40_mimotopes
50. https://casereports.bmj.com/content/2018/bcr-2018-225539.short
51. https://link.springer.com/article/10.1007/s10072-010-0353-y
52. https://jasn.asnjournals.org/content/13/9/2320.abstract
53. https://academic.oup.com/jnci/article/91/2/119/2549299
54. https://pubmed.ncbi.nlm.nih.gov/32266792/

55. https://pubmed.ncbi.nlm.nih.gov/28741088/
56. https://pubmed.ncbi.nlm.nih.gov/26728772/
57. https://www.nature.com/articles/cmi2017151
58. https://pubmed.ncbi.nlm.nih.gov/34957554/#:~:text=Recently%2C%20new%2Donset%20autoimmune%20phenomena,arthritis%20and%20systemic%20lupus%20erythematosus).
59. https://onlinelibrary.wiley.com/doi/full/10.1111/ene.15147
60. https://www.fda.gov/drugs/drug-interactions-labeling/preventable-adverse-drug-reactions-focus-drug-interactions

References for Point Number Eight

1. https://www.aapsonline.org/vaccines/mercinmed.pdf
2. https://www.autismspeaks.org/autism-statistics-asd
3. https://pubmed.ncbi.nlm.nih.gov/14595043/
4. https://bolenreport.com/wp-content/uploads/2016/04/Reference-10-Verstraeten-letter-to-Pediatrics-April-2004.pdf
5. https://childrenshealthdefense.org/news/vaccines-and-autism-is-the-science-really-settled/
6. https://pubmed.ncbi.nlm.nih.gov/24995277/
7. *The Environmental and Genetic Causes of Autism* by James Lyons-Weiler, PHD
8. https://pubmed.ncbi.nlm.nih.gov/9756729/
9. https://pubmed.ncbi.nlm.nih.gov/22015977/
10. https://pubmed.ncbi.nlm.nih.gov/23843785/
11. https://pubmed.ncbi.nlm.nih.gov/22290858/
12. https://pubmed.ncbi.nlm.nih.gov/21549155/
13. http://omsj.org/reports/tomljenovic%202011.pdf
14. https://pubmed.ncbi.nlm.nih.gov/17974154/
15. https://pubmed.ncbi.nlm.nih.gov/17454560/
16. https://pubmed.ncbi.nlm.nih.gov/21623535/
17. https://link.springer.com/article/10.1007/s10565-009-9124-z
18. https://pubmed.ncbi.nlm.nih.gov/12145534/
19. http://adventuresinautism.com/Hewitsonetal2010.pdf
20. https://pubmed.ncbi.nlm.nih.gov/21225508/
21. https://pubmed.ncbi.nlm.nih.gov/29329213/
22. https://www.tandfonline.com/doi/abs/10.1080/02772240701806501#

23. https://www.nature.com/articles/4001529
24. http://www.jpands.org/vol9no2/bradstreet.pdf
25. https://pubmed.ncbi.nlm.nih.gov/21623535/
26. https://pubmed.ncbi.nlm.nih.gov/16512356/
27. https://link.springer.com/article/10.1186/1742-2094-10-46
28. https://onlinelibrary.wiley.com/doi/abs/10.1002/ana.20315
29. https://www.ncbi.nlm.nih.gov/pmc/articles/PMC6027314/
30. https://pubmed.ncbi.nlm.nih.gov/23843785/
31. https://pubmed.ncbi.nlm.nih.gov/17454560/
32. https://pubmed.ncbi.nlm.nih.gov/16766480/
33. https://pubmed.ncbi.nlm.nih.gov/21058170/
34. https://pubmed.ncbi.nlm.nih.gov/18404135/
35. https://pubmed.ncbi.nlm.nih.gov/21623535/
36. https://www.ncbi.nlm.nih.gov/pmc/articles/PMC3774468/
37. https://pubmed.ncbi.nlm.nih.gov/18482737/
38. https://www.hindawi.com/journals/jt/2012/373678/
39. https://pubmed.ncbi.nlm.nih.gov/16273274/
40. https://www.ncbi.nlm.nih.gov/pubmed/29413113
41. https://www.ncbi.nlm.nih.gov/pubmed/29773196
42. https://asatonline.org/research-treatment/resources/topical-articles/autism-and-vaccines-the-evidence-to-date/
43. http://avoiceforchoice.org/wp-content/uploads/2015/12/STATEMENT-OF-WILLIAM-W.-THOMPSON-Ph.D.-REGARDING-THE-2004-ARTICLE-EXAMINING-THE-POSSIBILITY-OF-A-RELATIONSHIP-BETWEEN-MMR-VACCINE-AND-AUTISM.pdf
44. https://abcnews.go.com/Health/now-retracted-autism-study-viral/story?id=25248179
45. https://pubmed.ncbi.nlm.nih.gov/21785120/
46. https://www.nejm.org/doi/full/10.1056/nejmoa071434
47. https://childrenshealthdefense.org/wp-content/uploads/2016/11/Dr_BrianHooker_statement_regarding_Vaccine_Whistleblower_William_Thompson.pdf
48. https://thehill.com/blogs/pundits-blog/healthcare/301432-the-cdc-is-being-being-influenced-by-corporate-and-political
49. https://ahrp.org/former-merck-scientists-sue-merck-alleging-mmr-vaccine-efficacy-fraud/

50. https://pubmed.ncbi.nlm.nih.gov/18976924/
51. https://pubmed.ncbi.nlm.nih.gov/9481001/
52. https://pubmed.ncbi.nlm.nih.gov/28741088/
53. https://www.ninds.nih.gov/Disorders/All-Disorders/Encephalopathy-Information-Page#:~:text=The%20hallmark%20of%20encephalopathy%20is,and%20progressive%20loss%20of%20consciousness.
54. https://digitalcommons.pace.edu/pelr/vol28/iss2/6/
55. https://www.fda.gov/drugs/drug-interactions-labeling/preventable-adverse-drug-reactions-focus-drug-interactions
56. https://www.longdom.org/open-access/autism-is-an-acquired-cellular-detoxification-deficiency-syndrome-with-heterogeneous-genetic-predisposition-2165-7890-1000224.pdf
57. https://sharylattkisson.com/2023/07/dr-andrew-zimmermans-full-affidavit-on-alleged-link-between-vaccines-and-autism-that-u-s-govt-covered-up/
58. https://www.nlm.nih.gov/oet/ed/stats/02-400.html#:~:text=Temporal%20Precedence%20%2D%20The%20hypothesized%20cause,two%20variables%20regardless%20of%20causation.
59. https://www.npr.org/2008/03/07/87974932/case-stokes-debate-about-autism-vaccines

References for Point Number Nine

1. https://www.ncbi.nlm.nih.gov/pmc/articles/PMC4157320/
2. https://www.tandfonline.com/doi/abs/10.1080/02772240701806501
3. http://www.revahb.fr/Files/Other/Documents/Gallagher-HBV-vacc-Male-Neonates-and-Autism-2010.pdf
4. http://avoiceforchoice.org/wp-content/uploads/2015/12/STATEMENT-OF-WILLIAM-W.-THOMPSON-Ph.D.-REGARDING-THE-2004-ARTICLE-EXAMINING-THE-POSSIBILITY-OF-A-RELATIONSHIP-BETWEEN-MMR-VACCINE-AND-AUTISM.pdf
5. https://onlinelibrary.wiley.com/doi/full/10.1111/jjns.12252
6. https://www.sciencedirect.com/science/article/abs/pii/S0161475400900721

7. https://www.ncbi.nlm.nih.gov/pmc/articles/PMC5360569/
8. https://www.bmj.com/content/343/bmj.d5956.long
9. https://yale62.org/wp-content/uploads/2021/06/Verstraeten-Thomas-M.D.-et-al-CDC-1999.pdf
10. https://www.oatext.com/pdf/JTS-3-186.pdf
11. https://www.oatext.com/health-effects-in-vaccinated-versus-unvaccinated-children-with-covariates-for-breastfeeding-status-and-type-of-birth.php
12. https://www.sciencedirect.com/science/article/abs/pii/S0091674905000266
13. https://ijvtpr.com/index.php/IJVTPR/article/view/40?utm_source=substack&utm_medium=email

References for Point Number Ten

1. https://www.marinhealthcare.org/upload/public-meetings/2018-06-19-600-pm-mhd-community-health-seminar-vaccination/BRANCO_06192018_MGH%20Vaccine%20Presentation.pdf
2. https://www.chop.edu/centers-programs/vaccine-education-center/vaccine-history/developments-by-year
3. https://www.congress.gov/bill/99th-congress/house-bill/5546
4. https://www.cdc.gov/vaccines/schedules/hcp/imz/child-adolescent.html
5. https://www.pharmacytimes.com/view/new-vaccines-in-the-pipeline-2020
6. https://www.nih.gov/news-events/news-releases/autoimmunity-may-be-rising-united-states
7. https://www.autismspeaks.org/autism-statistics-asd
8. https://pubmed.ncbi.nlm.nih.gov/23733895/
9. https://waojournal.biomedcentral.com/articles/10.1186/1939-4551-7-12#:~:text=The%20prevalence%20of%20allergic%20diseases,greatest%20burden%20of%20these%20trends.
10. https://www.americashealthrankings.org/learn/reports/2019-annual-report/international-comparison
11. https://www.sciencedirect.com/science/article/abs/pii/S0022347607001850

12. https://link.springer.com/article/10.1186/s12199-020-00864-7
13. https://academic.oup.com/trstmh/article-abstract/109/1/77/1922615
14. https://pubmed.ncbi.nlm.nih.gov/20628439/
15. https://journals.sagepub.com/doi/abs/10.1177/0960327111407644
16. https://healthydogworkshop.com/wp-content/uploads/2019/05/javma2E20052E2272E1102-1.pdf
17. https://citeseerx.ist.psu.edu/viewdoc/download?doi=10.1.1.227.8653&rep=rep1&type=pdf
18. https://www.sciencedirect.com/science/article/abs/pii/S0022347697700568
19. https://pubmed.ncbi.nlm.nih.gov/22531966/
20. https://pubmed.ncbi.nlm.nih.gov/23338829/
21. https://www.oatext.com/pdf/JTS-3-186.pdf
22. https://www.oatext.com/health-effects-in-vaccinated-versus-unvaccinated-children-with-covariates-for-breastfeeding-status-and-type-of-birth.php
23. https://www.sciencedirect.com/science/article/abs/pii/S0091674905000266
24. https://www.pbs.org/wgbh/frontline/article/robert-w-sears-why-partial-vaccinations-may-be-an-answer/#:~:text=The%20CDC%20groups%20six%20vaccines,4%20months%20and%206%20months.
25. https://www.hhs.gov/immunization/who-and-when/infants-to-teens/index.html
26. https://www.immunology.org/public-information/bitesized-immunology/immune-development/neonatal-immunology

References for Point Number Eleven

1. https://www.thelancet.com/journals/lancet/article/PIIS0140-6736(97)11096-0/fulltext
2. https://briandeer.com/wakefield/royal-video.htm
3. https://briandeer.com/mmr/1998-vaccine-patent.pdf
4. https://patents.justia.com/assignee/centers-for-disease-control-and-prevention?page=10

5. https://www.cdc.gov/vaccines/imz-managers/guides-pubs/downloads/vacc_mandates_chptr13.pdf
6. https://www.upi.com/UPI-Investigates-The-vaccine-conflict/44221058841736/
7. https://issuu.com/wakefieldjusticefund
8. https://thehighwire.com/videos/the-most-important-interview-of-our-time-highwire-episode-91/
9. https://briandeer.com/mmr/lancet-deer-1.htm
10. https://www.thelancet.com/journals/lancet/article/PIIS0140-6736(97)11096-0/fulltext
11. https://www.historyofvaccines.org/content/blog/bmj-wakefield-paper-alleging-link-between-mmr-vaccine-and-autism-fraudulent
12. https://www.ncbi.nlm.nih.gov/pmc/articles/PMC3136032/
13. https://time.com/5175704/andrew-wakefield-vaccine-autism/
14. https://www.npr.org/sections/health-shots/2013/05/21/185801259/fifteen-years-after-a-vaccine-scare-a-measles-epidemic
15. https://www.gov.uk/government/publications/measles-deaths-by-age-group-from-1980-to-2013-ons-data/measles-notifications-and-deaths-in-england-and-wales-1940-to-2013
16. https://www.sciencedirect.com/science/article/abs/pii/001650859170014O
17. https://pubmed.ncbi.nlm.nih.gov/8492105/
18. https://www.thelancet.com/journals/lancet/article/PIIS0140-6736%2895%2990816-1/fulltext#%20
19. https://link.springer.com/article/10.1007/BF01211371
20. https://www.sciencedirect.com/science/article/abs/pii/S0002927000020414
21. https://link.springer.com/article/10.1023/A:1005443726670
22. https://onlinelibrary.wiley.com/doi/full/10.1046/j.1365-2036.2002.01206.x
23. https://www.sciencedirect.com/science/article/abs/pii/S1590865801800244
24. https://mp.bmj.com/content/55/2/84.long
25. https://www.sciencedirect.com/science/article/abs/pii/S0022347601922279

26. https://link.springer.com/article/10.1023/B:JO-CI.0000010427.05143.bb
27. https://link.springer.com/article/10.1007/s10875-004-6241-6
28. https://www.sciencedirect.com/science/article/abs/pii/S0165572805005394
29. https://pubmed.ncbi.nlm.nih.gov/28078206/
30. https://pubmed.ncbi.nlm.nih.gov/30747427/
31. https://journals.lww.com/eurojgh/Abstract/2020/03000/Environmental_exposures_and_the_risk_of.10.aspx
32. https://briandeer.com/mmr/lancet-retraction.pdf
33. https://www.theguardian.com/society/2012/mar/07/mmr-row-doctor-appeal
34. https://www.theguardian.com/science/2004/feb/26/thisweeks-sciencequestions1
35. https://www.nature.com/articles/479157a
36. https://www.bizpacreview.com/2022/01/16/doctor-loses-license-ordered-to-have-psych-eval-for-prescribing-ivermectin-sharing-covid-falsehoods-1189313/
37. https://www.latimes.com/local/lanow/la-me-sears-vaccine-20160909-snap-story.html
38. https://www.washingtonpost.com/local/md-politics/regulators-who-targeted-anti-vaccine-doctor-may-pay-millions-for-humiliating-him/2018/02/03/b63ea6dc-faf8-11e7-ad8c-ecbb62019393_story.html
39. https://www.phoenixnewtimes.com/news/anti-vaccination-doctor-under-investigation-by-arizona-medical-board-6627760
40. https://www.medpagetoday.com/special-reports/exclusives/93566
41. https://www.forbes.com/sites/tarahaelle/2019/06/21/dr-bob-sears-accused-of-issuing-invalid-vaccine-medical-exemptions-again/?sh=ba8675d447a4
42. https://www.wsj.com/articles/youtube-the-who-and-censoring-medical-speech-11600375547
43. https://www.jccf.ca/surgeon-fired-by-college-of-medicine-for-voicing-safety-concerns-about-covid-shots-for-children/
44. https://www.youtube.com/watch?v=Bz-c1Vst9fs

45. https://www.fiercehealthcare.com/practices/physician-groups-back-doctors-freedom-to-speak-out-about-coronavirus-conditions
46. https://historyofvaccines.org/vaccines-101/misconceptions-about-vaccines/history-anti-vaccination-movements

References for Point Number Twelve

1. https://bshm.org.uk/herd-immunity-whats-in-a-name/
2. https://academic.oup.com/cid/article/52/7/911/299077?fbclid=IwAR2ddU3JbjJxoHYbJal9nqz-KV39sCmd_3r46rWKLKW37ETY6c2uWk6A67ZQ
3. https://physics.mcmaster.ca/~higgsp/756/Fox_1971.pdf
4. https://www.sciencedirect.com/science/article/pii/S1877282X10000299
5. https://www.publichealth.columbia.edu/public-health-now/news/relationship-between-vaccines-and-herd-immunity
6. https://www.cdc.gov/vaccines/imz-managers/guides-pubs/downloads/vacc_mandates_chptr13.pdf
7. https://www.cdc.gov/mmwr/volumes/69/wr/mm6942a1.htm
8. https://www.cdc.gov/mmwr/volumes/67/wr/mm6740a4.htm
9. http://www.tetyanaobukhanych.com/herd_immunity.html
10. https://www.cdc.gov/mmwr/volumes/68/wr/mm6841e2.htm
11. https://www.statista.com/statistics/385577/mmr-vaccination-rate-among-us-children-aged-19-35-months/
12. https://www.medicine.wisc.edu/sites/default/files/reemergence_of_measles_safdar.pdf
13. https://www.nature.com/articles/318323a0.pdf?origin=ppub
14. https://jamanetwork.com/journals/jamainternalmedicine/article-abstract/619215
15. https://academic.oup.com/cid/article/58/9/1205/2895266?login=true
16. https://pubmed.ncbi.nlm.nih.gov/1861205/
17. https://jamanetwork.com/journals/jamapediatrics/article-abstract/517604
18. https://pubmed.ncbi.nlm.nih.gov/14993534/#:~:text=Conclusions%3A%20A%20chickenpox%20outbreak%20occurred,vaccination%20may%20deserve%20additional%20consideration.

19. https://www.cdc.gov/pertussis/about/faqs.html
20. https://www.nejm.org/doi/full/10.1056/NEJM197301112880204
21. https://www.tandfonline.com/doi/full/10.1080/21645515.2015.1093263
22. https://journals.lww.com/pidj/Fulltext/2013/07000/Primary_Versus_Secondary_Failure_After_Varicella.21.aspx#:~:text=Primary%20vaccine%20failure%20could%20be,waning%20of%20immunity%20over%20time.
23. https://academic.oup.com/jid/article/181/2/725/825708
24. https://www.ncbi.nlm.nih.gov/books/NBK8149/
25. https://emedicine.medscape.com/article/217146-overview#showall
26. https://www.ncbi.nlm.nih.gov/pmc/articles/PMC228449/pdf/332485.pdf
27. https://www.ncbi.nlm.nih.gov/pmc/articles/PMC8158893/
28. https://www.cdc.gov/nchs/products/databriefs/db281.htm
29. https://www.statista.com/statistics/1239490/us-adults-who-received-clinical-preventive-services/
30. https://www.cdc.gov/vaccines/imz-managers/coverage/adultvaxview/pubs-resources/NHIS-2016.html
31. https://www.tandfonline.com/doi/full/10.4161/21645515.2014.982998
32. https://www.science.org/content/article/how-long-do-vaccines-last-surprising-answers-may-help-protect-people-longer
33. Moralization of Covid-19 health response: Asymmetry in tolerance for human costs - ScienceDirect

References for Point Number Thirteen

1. https://www.pewresearch.org/science/2018/11/19/public-perspectives-on-food-risks/
2. https://www.foodnavigator-usa.com/Article/2021/06/18/IFIC-Americans-are-paying-more-attention-to-ingredients-looking-for-clean-natural-options
3. https://www.statista.com/statistics/244393/share-of-organic-sales-in-the-united-states/

4. https://www.statista.com/statistics/223413/public-concern-about-air-pollution-in-the-us/
5. https://progressivegrocer.com/consumers-manufacturers-seek-cleaner-clean
6. https://www.globenewswire.com/news-release/2020/06/23/2052153/0/en/Global-Green-Cleaning-Products-Market-Thriving-Worldwide-Trends-Analysis-and-Forecast-2019-2029-PMI.html
7. https://pubmed.ncbi.nlm.nih.gov/22235057/
8. https://pubmed.ncbi.nlm.nih.gov/23932735/
9. https://www.frontiersin.org/articles/10.3389/fneur.2015.00004/ful
10. https://www.ncbi.nlm.nih.gov/pmc/articles/PMC5214894/#:~:text=Contact%20allergy%20to%20aluminium%20was,4%2C%207%2C%209).
11. https://pubmed.ncbi.nlm.nih.gov/29413113/#:~:text=The%20aluminium%20content%20of%20brain%20tissue%20in%20autism%20was%20consistently,temporal%20and%20parietal%20lobes%20respectively.
12. https://www.researchgate.net/publication/319216249_HEAVY_METAL_OVERLOAD_IN_AUTISTIC_CHILDREN
13. https://pubmed.ncbi.nlm.nih.gov/26265215/
14. https://aacijournal.biomedcentral.com/articles/10.1186/s13223-018-0305-2
15. https://www.sciencedirect.com/topics/medicine-and-dentistry/framycetin
16. https://www.cdc.gov/vaccines/pubs/pinkbook/downloads/appendices/B/excipient-table-2.pdf
17. https://www.longdom.org/open-access/evidence-that-food-proteins-in-vaccines-cause-the-development-of-food-allergies-and-its-implications-for-vaccine-policy-12461.html
18. https://pubmed.ncbi.nlm.nih.gov/26103708/
19. https://www.jacionline.org/article/S0091-6749(07)02379-2/fulltext#%20
20. https://pubmed.ncbi.nlm.nih.gov/9345669/
21. https://www.sciencedirect.com/science/article/abs/pii/S0091674905000266

22. https://pubmed.ncbi.nlm.nih.gov/10714532/
23. https://erj.ersjournals.com/content/20/2/403.short
24. https://onlinelibrary.wiley.com/doi/abs/10.1034/j.1398-9995.1999.00763.x
25. https://hero.epa.gov/hero/index.cfm/reference/details/reference_id/4320
26. https://www.ncbi.nlm.nih.gov/pmc/articles/PMC5938543/
27. https://www.ncbi.nlm.nih.gov/pmc/articles/PMC6952072/
28. https://pubs.rsc.org/en/content/articlehtml/2017/ra/c6ra27242h
29. https://www.sciencedirect.com/science/article/abs/pii/0378517389902664
30. https://link.springer.com/article/10.1023/A:1018983904537
31. https://www.sciencedirect.com/science/article/abs/pii/S014296120300855X
32. https://link.springer.com/article/10.1023/A:1018947208597
33. https://link.springer.com/article/10.1023/A:1012098005098
34. https://www.ncbi.nlm.nih.gov/pmc/articles/PMC3061435/
35. https://casereports.bmj.com/content/2012/bcr.02.2012.5797.short
36. https://www.who.int/news-room/questions-and-answers/item/mercury-health
37. https://www.ncbi.nlm.nih.gov/pmc/articles/PMC3600517/#:~:text=Mercuric%20chloride%20(HgCl2)%20did,modify%20Jurkat%20T%20cell%20viability.
38. https://pubmed.ncbi.nlm.nih.gov/21350943/
39. https://www.sciencedirect.com/science/article/abs/pii/S0940299308001206

References for Point Number Fourteen

1. https://www.cdc.gov/chickenpox/hcp/index.html
2. https://www.drugtopics.com/view/shingles-complications-elderly
3. https://elifesciences.org/articles/07116
4. https://www.tandfonline.com/doi/full/10.1080/21645515.2018.1546525
5. https://link.springer.com/article/10.1006/bulm.1999.0126

6. https://link.springer.com/article/10.1186/1471-2458-5-68/
7. https://www.sciencedirect.com/science/article/abs/pii/S0163445302909886
8. https://journals.lww.com/pidj/fulltext/2009/11000/The_Incidence_and_Clinical_Characteristics_of.4.aspx
9. https://journals.plos.org/plosone/article?id=10.1371/journal.pone.0060732
10. https://europepmc.org/backend/ptpmcrender.fcgi?accid=PMC2563790&blobtype=pdf
11. https://www.tandfonline.com/doi/full/10.4161/hv.34426
12. https://www.news-medical.net/news/2005/09/01/12896.aspx
13. https://www.jscimedcentral.com/Pathology/pathology-6-1133.pdf
14. https://www.sciencedirect.com/science/article/pii/S1098301520344478
15. https://rickjaffeesq.com/wp-content/uploads/2021/02/r18hs017045-lazarus-final-report-20116.pdf
16. https://pubmed.ncbi.nlm.nih.gov/10979114/
17. https://www.proclinical.com/blogs/2016-9/top-selling-vaccines-in-pharmaceutical-history
18. https://www.biopharmadive.com/news/merck-shinges-vaccine-lawsuits-zostavax/438125/

References for Point Number Fifteen

1. https://www.immunize.org/vaccines/vis/about-vis/
2. https://www.immunize.org/wp-content/uploads/vis/flu_inactive.pdf
3. https://www.who.int/news-room/fact-sheets/detail/influenza-(seasonal)#:~:text=There%20are%20around%20a%20billion,650%20000%20respiratory%20deaths%20annually
4. https://pubmed.ncbi.nlm.nih.gov/6247520/
5. https://pubmed.ncbi.nlm.nih.gov/1851395/
6. https://pubmed.ncbi.nlm.nih.gov/19730016/
7. https://www.cdc.gov/flu/highrisk/pregnant.htm
8. https://www.path.org/our-impact/articles/why-are-pregnant-people-left-out-vaccine-research/

9. https://www.npr.org/2020/12/11/945196602/pregnant-people-havent-been-part-of-vaccine-trials-should-they-get-the-vaccine
10. https://www.sciencedirect.com/science/article/abs/pii/S0264410X23012598
11. https://www.sciencedirect.com/science/article/abs/pii/S0264410X17308666
12. https://onlinelibrary.wiley.com/doi/full/10.1111/irv.12897
13. https://pubmed.ncbi.nlm.nih.gov/23023030/
14. https://jamanetwork.com/journals/jamainternalmedicine/fullarticle/486407#:~:text=Background%20Observational%20studies%20report%20that,1980%20to%2065%25%20in%202001.
15. https://www.cidrap.umn.edu/influenza-vaccines/another-study-shows-limited-flu-vaccine-benefits-seniors
16. https://www.ncbi.nlm.nih.gov/pmc/articles/PMC2271825/
17. https://www.cdc.gov/flu/vaccines-work/past-seasons-estimates.html
18. https://www.ncbi.nlm.nih.gov/pmc/articles/PMC1953433/?page=1
19. https://publications.aap.org/pediatrics/article-abstract/78/4/728/79499/Varicella-Complications-and-Costs
20. https://www.cdc.gov/vaccines/hcp/vis/vis-statements/varicella.pdf
21. https://academic.oup.com/aje/article/183/8/765/1739793?login=false
22. https://pubmed.ncbi.nlm.nih.gov/16126614/
23. https://pubmed.ncbi.nlm.nih.gov/12057605/
24. https://www.ncbi.nlm.nih.gov/books/NBK441824/
25. https://pubmed.ncbi.nlm.nih.gov/22423127/
26. https://pubmed.ncbi.nlm.nih.gov/25560446/
27. https://pubmed.ncbi.nlm.nih.gov/11740314/
28. https://pubmed.ncbi.nlm.nih.gov/24216286/
29. https://pubmed.ncbi.nlm.nih.gov/7645380/
30. https://academic.oup.com/cid/article/54/12/1730/452864
31. https://www.cdc.gov/mmwr/preview/mmwrhtml/00020038.htm
32. https://academic.oup.com/cid/article/70/1/152/5525423?login=false

33. https://www.cdc.gov/vaccines/hcp/vis/vis-statements/dtap.pdf
34. https://pubmed.ncbi.nlm.nih.gov/3835080/
35. https://pubmed.ncbi.nlm.nih.gov/18670/
36. https://pubmed.ncbi.nlm.nih.gov/240337/
37. https://www.thelancet.com/journals/ebiom/article/PIIS2352-3964(17)30046-4/fulltext
38. https://biomedres.us/pdfs/BJSTR.MS.ID.000528.pdf
39. https://pubmed.ncbi.nlm.nih.gov/18976924/
40. https://www.cdc.gov/mmwr/preview/MMWRhtml/00033405.htm
41. https://www.hhs.gov/hepatitis/learn-about-viral-hepatitis/hepatitis-b-basics/index.html#:~:text=In%20the%20United%20States%2C%20rates,crisis%20and%20other%20drug%20use.
42. https://www.mdpi.com/2076-0817/9/6/432#:~:text=cohorts%20%5B9%5D.-,People%20who%20inject%20drugs%20(PWID)%20and%20female%20sex%20workers%20(,including%20HIV%2C%20HCV%20and%20HBV.
43. https://pubmed.ncbi.nlm.nih.gov/21691704/
44. https://pubmed.ncbi.nlm.nih.gov/12397738/
45. https://pubmed.ncbi.nlm.nih.gov/10230847/
46. https://www.sciencedirect.com/science/article/abs/pii/S104346661830190X?via%3Dihub
47. https://www.sciencedirect.com/science/article/abs/pii/S0306453016305145?via%3Dihub
48. https://pubmed.ncbi.nlm.nih.gov/22249285/
49. https://www.sciencedirect.com/science/article/abs/pii/S0264410X05003506?via%3Dihub
50. https://pubmed.ncbi.nlm.nih.gov/20207367/
51. https://onlinelibrary.wiley.com/doi/10.1155/2016/2401809
52. https://pubmed.ncbi.nlm.nih.gov/25427994/
53. https://pubmed.ncbi.nlm.nih.gov/18725327/
54. https://pubmed.ncbi.nlm.nih.gov/19730016/

References for Point Number Sixteen

1. https://effectiviology.com/credentials-fallacy/#:~:text=In%20addition%2C%20the%20credentials%20fallacy,credentials%20are%20relevant%20or%20necessary.

2. https://www.ajpmfocus.org/article/S2773-0654(23)00115-3/fulltext
3. https://thevaccinereaction.org/2018/07/what-doctors-learn-in-medical-school-about-vaccines/#_edn2
4. https://static1.squarespace.com/static/56d36e9d86db43f4f-77637c1/t/5d71050e89e6870001d106cd/1567687985997/Blay-lock+on+vaccines+and+the+developing+brain.pdf
5. https://scentses4d.wordpress.com/2019/04/29/medical-doc-tors-and-phds-speak-out-against-vaccinations/
6. https://wvpublic.org/story/health-science/lawmakers-hear-from-all-sides-of-vaccine-debate/
7. https://www.informedchoicewa.org/20-problems-vaccine-sci-ence/
8. https://vaccinationinformationnetwork.com/jim-mee-han-md-to-all-pediatricians/?fbclid=IwAR1d6NuhYXD3xS_uF-NJf1vF1r2aJE4lUBOz_FCk_Y2UoaS70_hj-E0b5eCA
9. https://www.uscjournal.com/authors/peter-mccullough
10. https://www.independent.org/person/robert-w-malone-m-d-m-s/
11. https://www.politifact.com/article/2022/jan/06/who-robert-malone-joe-rogans-guest-was-vaccine-sci/

References for Point Number Seventeen

1. https://www.ncsl.org/health/states-with-religious-and-philo-sophical-exemptions-from-school-immunization-requirements
2. https://www.ksby.com/news/california-news/a-new-ca-bill-could-allow-12-to-17-year-olds-to-get-vaccinated-without-paren-tal-consent
3. https://fee.org/articles/californias-war-on-homeschoolers/
4. https://www.californiahomeschool.net/how-to-homeschool/legal-options/
5. https://gvwire.com/2018/03/23/battle-isnt-over-for-homes-choolers-new-regulations-ahead/
6. https://www.cdc.gov/mmwr/volumes/69/wr/mm6942a1.htm
7. https://www.usnews.com/news/national-news/arti-cles/2019-01-16/who-names-vaccine-hesitancy-as-top-world-threat-in-2019

8. https://www.ajmc.com/view/a-timeline-of-covid19-developments-in-2020
9. https://nypost.com/2021/02/19/white-house-working-with-social-media-to-silence-anti-vaxxers/?utm_source=facebook&utm_medium=news_tab&utm_content=algorithm&fbclid=IwAR2v6-yrYWyiLmTwbmhs_gPyg4WclVS1r9xsNOl-YC0Pl0NXPBQZb3e5Kwc
10. https://www.bmj.com/content/371/bmj.m4425
11. https://www.ncbi.nlm.nih.gov/pmc/articles/PMC7717882/
12. https://www.forbes.com/sites/robertpearl/2020/09/22/3-misleading-dangerous-coronavirus-statistics/?sh=7b432cd67169
13. https://www.cnn.com/asia/live-news/coronavirus-outbreak-02-19-20-intl-hnk/index.html
14. https://pubmed.ncbi.nlm.nih.gov/36341800/
15. https://www.who.int/news-room/fact-sheets/detail/influenza-(seasonal)#:~:text=There%20are%20around%20a%20billion,650%20000%20respiratory%20deaths%20annually.
16. https://www.kusi.com/cdc-director-75-of-covid-deaths-occurred-in-people-with-at-least-four-comorbidities/
17. https://link.springer.com/article/10.1007/s42399-020-00363-4
18. https://link.springer.com/article/10.1007/s40520-020-01664-3
19. https://journals.plos.org/plosone/article?id=10.1371/journal.pone.0241824
20. https://www.mayoclinic.org/diseases-conditions/coronavirus/in-depth/coronavirus-who-is-at-risk/art-20483301#:~:text=Older%20age,highest%20risk%20of%20serious%20symptoms.
21. https://www.ncbi.nlm.nih.gov/pmc/articles/PMC8479338/#:~:text=However%2C%20older%20age%20appears%20to,year%2Dolds%20%5B13%5D.
22. https://www.cdc.gov/mmwr/volumes/70/wr/mm7003e1.htm
23. https://adc.bmj.com/content/106/5/429
24. https://jamanetwork.com/journals/jamanetworkopen/fullarticle/2777314
25. https://www.rockefeller.edu/news/28008-gene-hunt-explain-young-healthy-people-die-covid-19/
26. https://www.washingtonexaminer.com/news/coronavirus-death-certificates-minnesota-inflated

27. https://www.washingtonpost.com/investigations/which-deaths-count-toward-the-covid-19-death-toll-it-depends-on-the-state/2020/04/16/bca84ae0-7991-11ea-a130-df573469f094_story.html
28. https://www.latimes.com/business/story/2020-10-22/death-certificates-covid-coronavirus-infections
29. https://www.rev.com/blog/transcripts/donald-trump-coronavirus-task-force-briefing-april-7
30. https://www.aamc.org/news-insights/how-are-covid-19-deaths-counted-it-s-complicated
31. https://www.usatoday.com/story/news/factcheck/2020/04/24/fact-check-medicare-hospitals-paid-more-covid-19-patients-coronavirus/3000638001/
32. https://www.cnn.com/2020/02/29/health/face-masks-coronavirus-surgeon-general-trnd/index.html
33. https://www.factcheck.org/2020/05/outdated-fauci-video-on-face-masks-shared-out-of-context/
34. https://edition.cnn.com/2020/05/27/politics/fauci-coronavirus-wear-masks-cnntv/index.html
35. https://www.cnbc.com/2020/06/05/dr-anthony-fauci-says-americans-who-dont-wear-masks-may-propagate-the-spread-of-infection.html
36. https://www.cnn.com/2020/03/30/world/coronavirus-who-masks-recommendation-trnd/index.html
37. https://www.ecdc.europa.eu/sites/default/files/documents/covid-19-face-masks-community-first-update.pdf
38. https://www.nbcnews.com/health/health-news/do-you-need-mask-science-hasn-t-changed-public-guidance-n1173006
39. https://www.who.int/publications/i/item/non-pharmaceutical-public-health-measuresfor-mitigating-the-risk-and-impact-of-epidemic-and-pandemic-influenza
40. https://www.ncbi.nlm.nih.gov/pmc/articles/PMC7357397/
41. https://www.fda.gov/medical-devices/personal-protective-equipment-infection-control/n95-respirat ors-surgical-masks-face-masks-and-barrier-face-coverings

42. https://www.fda.gov/medical-devices/personal-protective-equipment-infection-control/n95-respirators-surgical-masks-face-masks-and-barrier-face-coverings
43. https://bmjopen.bmj.com/content/5/4/e006577
44. https://www.acpjournals.org/doi/10.7326/M20-6817
45. https://wwwnc.cdc.gov/eid/article/26/5/19-0994_article
46. https://journals.plos.org/plosone/article?id=10.1371/journal.pone.0240287
47. https://www.cebm.net/covid-19/masking-lack-of-evidence-with-politics/
48. https://www.cochrane.org/CD006207/ARI_do-physical-measures-such-hand-washing-or-wearing-masks-stop-or-slow-down-spread-respiratory-viruses
49. https://escipub.com/irjph-2021-08-1005/
50. https://adc.bmj.com/content/108/2/131
51. https://www.nejm.org/doi/full/10.1056/NEJMp2006372
52. https://www.nejm.org/doi/full/10.1056/NEJMp2006372
53. https://www.cdc.gov/mmwr/volumes/69/wr/pdfs/mm6936-H.pdf
54. https://www.who.int/publications/i/item/advice-on-the-use-of-masks-in-the-community-during-home-care-and-in-healthcare-settings-in-the-context-of-the-novel-coronavirus-(2019-ncov)-outbreak
55. https://www.psycharchives.org/en/item/128fbeac-00e0-44bd-840e-e390594cd8de
56. https://www.medrxiv.org/content/10.1101/2022.05.10.22274813v1
57. https://www.fh-muenster.de/gesundheit/forschung/forschungsprojekte/moeglichkeiten-und-grenzen-der-eigenverantwortlichen-wiederverwendung-von-ffp2-masken-im-privatgebrauch/index.php
58. https://adc.bmj.com/content/109/3/e1
59. https://www.thelancet.com/journals/lanres/article/PIIS2213-2600(20)30323-4/fulltext
60. https://www.nature.com/articles/534024a
61. https://www.sciencedirect.com/science/article/pii/S0360132304003038

62. https://cognitiveresearchjournal.springeropen.com/articles/10.1186/s41235-022-00360-2
63. https://www.mdpi.com/2075-1729/11/11/1188
64. https://link.springer.com/article/10.1007/s00787-021-01924-1
65. https://journals.sagepub.com/doi/pdf/10.1177/0253717620982514
66. https://jamanetwork.com/journals/jamapediatrics/article-abstract/2788076
67. https://www.nytimes.com/2020/02/17/business/media/coronavirus-tom-cotton-china.html
68. https://jameslyonsweiler.com/2020/02/02/moderately-strong-confirmation-of-a-laboratory-origin-of-2019-ncov/
69. https://pmc.ncbi.nlm.nih.gov/articles/PMC7144200/
70. https://www.wsj.com/articles/covid-origin-china-lab-leak-807b7b0a
71. https://www.wsj.com/articles/fbi-director-says-covid-pandemic-likely-caused-by-chinese-lab-leak-13a5e69b
72. https://www.ncbi.nlm.nih.gov/pmc/articles/PMC7091063/
73. https://ard.bmj.com/content/77/1/98.abstract
74. https://link.springer.com/article/10.1007/s10654-022-00891-4
75. https://www.drugtargetreview.com/news/59414/ivermectin-shows-activity-against-covid-19-in-cell-cultures/
76. https://www.ncbi.nlm.nih.gov/pmc/articles/PMC7434458/
77. https://c19ivm.org/meta.html
78. https://www.ncbi.nlm.nih.gov/pmc/articles/PMC3043740/
79. https://www.fox35orlando.com/news/stop-it-fda-warns-ivermectin-is-not-a-covid-19-treatment-drug
80. https://www.merck.com/news/merck-statement-on-ivermectin-use-during-the-covid-19-pandemic/
81. https://thehighwire.com/ark-videos/former-w-h-o-consultant-exposes-takedown-of-ivermectin/
82. https://www.fda.gov/emergency-preparedness-and-response/mcm-legal-regulatory-and-policy-framework/emergency-use-authorization

83. https://www.somo.nl/big-pharma-raked-in-usd-90-billion-in-profits-with-covid-19-vaccines/#:~:text=Pharma's%20pandemic%20profits,-Pharma%20profits%20from&text=Pfizer%-20alone%20generated%20USD%2035,Sinovac%20pocketed%20USD%2015%20billion.
84. https://www.healthaffairs.org/content/forefront/government-produced-covid-19-vaccine-success
85. https://time.com/6092368/americas-frontline-doctors-covid-19-misinformation/
86. https://www.unmc.edu/healthsecurity/transmission/2024/08/14/doctors-accused-of-spreading-misinformation-lose-certifications/
87. https://www.jccf.ca/surgeon-fired-by-college-of-medicine-for-voicing-safety-concerns-about-covid-shots-for-children/
88. https://freedomhouse.org/report/report-sub-page/2020/information-isolation-censoring-covid-19-outbreak
89. https://www.beckershospitalreview.com/digital-marketing/physicians-who-post-covid-19-vaccine-misinformation-may-lose-license-medical-panel-says.html
90. https://www.glamour.com/story/anti-vaxx-celebrities-cant-stop-telling-on-themselves
91. https://www.factcheck.org/2024/02/scicheck-review-article-by-misinformation-spreaders-misleads-about-mrna-covid-19-vaccines/
92. https://principia-scientific.com/dr-jessica-rose-unloads-on-fda-advisory-panel/
93. https://www.beckershospitalreview.com/healthcare-information-technology/they-re-killing-people-biden-sounds-off-on-covid-19-misinformation-on-facebook.html
94. https://www.medscape.com/viewarticle/977677?src=wnl_newsalrt_220721_MSCPEDIT_Biden-Covid&uac=442068EV&impID=4449379
95. https://www.nih.gov/news-events/news-releases/niaid-director-fauci-tests-positive-covid-19
96. https://www.medrxiv.org/content/10.1101/2022.12.17.22283625v1

97. https://openvaers.com/covid-data
98. https://thehighwire.com/ark-videos/the-vaers-expose/
99. https://www.military.com/daily-news/2021/04/27/cdc-says-it-has-seen-no-signals-linking-covid-vaccines-and-myocarditis.html
100. https://jamanetwork.com/journals/jama/fullarticle/2788346
101. https://pubmed.ncbi.nlm.nih.gov/34957554/#:~:text=Recently%2C%20new%2Donset%20autoimmune%20phenomena,arthritis%20and%20systemic%20lupus%20erythematosus
102. https://www.ncbi.nlm.nih.gov/pmc/articles/PMC8242388/
103. https://onlinelibrary.wiley.com/doi/full/10.1111/ene.15147
104. https://www.tandfonline.com/doi/abs/10.1080/09273948.2021.1976221
105. https://onlinelibrary.wiley.com/doi/abs/10.1111/ane.13417
106. https://www.medrxiv.org/content/10.1101/2023.11.15.23298565v1
107. https://ijvtpr.com/index.php/IJVTPR/article/view/23
108. https://www.sciencedirect.com/science/article/pii/S0306987723000117
109. https://www.authorea.com/doi/full/10.22541/au.166203678.82079667
110. https://onlinelibrary.wiley.com/doi/full/10.1002/prca.202300048
111. https://doi.org/10.3390/microorganisms12071343
112. https://oversight.house.gov/wp-content/uploads/2024/12/2024.12.04-SSCP-FINAL-REPORT-ANS.pdf

About the Author

Dr. Michael Nichols is a chiropractor and functional nutritionist with over 25 years of clinical experience helping individuals and families achieve lasting health through natural, root-cause approaches. He is a Certified Personal Trainer, Certified Health Coach, Massage Therapist, and holds a Fellowship with the International Pediatric Chiropractic Association (ICPA).

In addition to his clinical work, Dr. Nichols has spent more than 20 years teaching anatomy, physiology, and pathophysiology to future healthcare professionals. A dynamic speaker and educator, he is also the host of The Flipside with Dr. Michael Nichols podcast, where he challenges conventional health perspectives and shares practical strategies for living well.

www.ingramcontent.com/pod-product-compliance
Lightning Source LLC
LaVergne TN
LVHW020509100826
845148LV00003B/729

* 9 7 9 8 2 1 8 8 7 7 3 1 6 *